Angela Hunt and
Laura Calenberg

Beauty
From the
Inside
Out

Professional
Secrets from
Top Models!

Hunt Haven

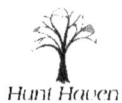

ISBN: 0615881726

ISBN 13: 978-0615881720

For my husband, Jeff, who has challenged me to concentrate on inner beauty and be the best I can be!

—Laura

For my daughter, Taryn, who is beautiful inside and out!

—Angie

CONTENTS

INTRODUCTION

If you asked a thousand different people to define *beautiful,* you'd probably get a thousand different answers. Beauty is found in so many places: in the glow from a new mother's face; the soft, tender face of a great-grandmother; the hush of a lake at sunset. Beauty is in a small child's laugh, the strong hands of a working man, and a young girl's smile.

Beauty can be found anywhere. You can even find it in yourself. You may not think of yourself as beautiful. Okay, perhaps. Passable, maybe. You might even think of yourself as ugly.

But beauty is found in many places. It's in your love for your parents, your smile for a friend, the offer of your hand to someone who needs help.

In his song "Picture Perfect," Michael W. Smith sings about a girl who puts her hair up and applies makeup to try to match the flawless faces of magazine covers. "Gaze in the mirror," he sings, "you want the glamour and the grace of a movie star — but I like you the way you are!"*

> You, girl
> You don't have to be picture perfect
> To be in my world....
> You're tender, you're tactful
> Girl, you're a natural
> You possess a heart that's true
> That's what I like about you!

1

ANGELA HUNT and LAURA CALENBERG

One in a million, yeah, that's given
There's a beauty inside of you
And it shows on the outside too.[1]

You can have the kind of beauty Michael W. Smith sings about. Beauty can be found *your* eyes, *your* smile, *your* form. You can be beautiful, the best you can be. Let us show you how.

---

[1] From "Picture Perfect" by Michael W. Smith and Wayne Kirkpatrick on the Reunion album "Change Your World." © 1992 O'Ryan Music, Inc. (ASCAP)/Emily Boothe, Inc. (BMI)/Magic Beans Music (BMI). Administered by Reunion Music Group. Used by permission.

1

HAIR, YOUR CROWNING GLORY

Do you hate your hair? Krista Marcy, a top model, once hated her naturally curly hair. She says:

> I hated my curly hair in high school. I'd spend hours trying to straighten it. But I've learned that if you use what God gave you and make the best of it, you'll receive compliments. I realized years later that people were actually paying hundreds of dollars to have the curly look that I had naturally. Ironically, my first major New York modeling job was for hair products.

Martin Luther once said, "The hair is the finest ornament women have."[1] Whether or not he was right, one of the first things people notice about you is your hair. Whether you wear it short, long, or in between, your hair says a great deal about how you feel about yourself.

What Is Hair?

A single hair is composed of three distinct layers. The outermost layer, the *cuticle*, is composed of hard flat scales that overlap like the shingles of a roof. These overlapping scales allow the hair to bend and twist without breaking. When hair is in good condition, the scales of the cuticle lie flat and smooth on the hair shaft. They reflect light and the hair shines. When hair is damaged or unhealthy, these protective scales break off and the resulting ragged edges leave the hair dull, drab, and lifeless.

The second layer of hair is the *cortex*. This fibrous inner core that gives hair strength, elasticity, and pliability makes up about 80 percent of the hail's bulk. The cortex produces pigment that results in hair color, and also determines the direction of growth, size, and diameter of strands of hair, hair texture, and quality.

The innermost layer of the hair, lying deep within the cortex, is the *medulla*. Its function is unknown.

Let's take a moment to test your hair. Pluck a single hair from your head and pull it firmly from both ends without breaking it. Examine it carefully. Does it shine? Now stretch it. Strong, healthy hair will stretch up to 25 percent of its length before it finally breaks. Dry or brittle hair will snap almost immediately.

Now run your fingers through your hair. Does it feel smooth and alive? It might, but the hair you can actually comb is dead. The living part of your hair is embedded beneath your scalp. If you want to help your hair, you must begin by improving the hair that is alive and growing.

You have between 90,000 and 140,000 hairs on your head— only God knows exactly how many. Each of those hairs grows about half an inch each month, but your hair grows fastest when you are between the ages of fifteen and twenty-five. Hair grows faster in summer than in winter, and faster at night than in the daytime.

Hair grows in cycles, and each individual hair is on its own timetable. A single hair will grow for a certain amount of time, usually between two to five years. Whenever this growing stage is complete, the hair stops growing for a week or two, then the hair rests and the old hair is pushed out and the cycle begins again.

If hair grows only for a few years and then falls out, how can some people grow their hair to their ankles? Angie's hairdresser, Bill Baker, explained that some people have hair cycles that continue up to ten years. The singer Crystal Gayle, whose hair is down to her ankles, probably has a twelve-year growth cycle. But whenever the cycle is done, the hair falls out and a new one replaces it. Fortunately, not all hairs are on the same "schedule," so there are always lots of other hairs around to fill in. That's why it's normal to have a certain amount of hair loss every day. Unless your hair falls out in clumps, you shouldn't worry about it.

If you want to nourish your hair, concentrate first on the hair that's still alive—the part of hair beneath your scalp, growing inside the hair follicle. Down inside the dermis, the layer of skin beneath the epidermis, is the papilla, a small bud at the base of each hair follicle. The hair root is formed in the papilla and is attached over it.

Small blood vessels carry the ingredients necessary for hair growth to the papilla, where vitamins, minerals, and water are changed into keratin, the tough substance of which hair and nails are composed. Keratin is a complex combination of amino acids, ten of which cannot be manufactured by the body alone. If you want healthy hair, you've got to eat healthy foods. You need foods containing protein, magnesium, folic acid, biotin, vitamin B-6, and zinc.

Diet for Beautiful Hair
Protein is found in meats, cheeses, eggs, fish, milk, tofu, yogurt, and peanut butter. You're probably eating plenty of protein already; in fact, most Americans consume too much. You only need two or three servings of protein food per day.

Magnesium, folic acid, biotin, and *vitamin B-6* are important for hair. You can find all or most of these ingredients in molasses, sunflower seeds, wheat germ, nuts, soybeans, brown rice, spinach, bananas, cheese, tuna, and potatoes.

Zinc is important for hair health, and it also makes a big difference if you have acne. Too little zinc can cause your skin to turn rough and your hair to fall out. Zinc is found in grain and wheat products, so choose whole wheat bread instead of white bread for maximum beauty and health benefits.

Water is the most important ingredient you can put into your body. We'll talk more about this later, but you should drink at least eight glasses of water each day.

By the way, one of the surest ways to wreck your hair is to go on a crash diet. If you go on a sudden starvation diet, your hair will broadcast the news to the world by its dull, scruffy appearance. It may even begin to fall out in clumps.

Facts and Fiction
The less you shampoo your hair, the healthier it will be.

Dirty hair is neither pretty nor healthy, and shampooing every day will not weaken your hair. Practically all modern shampoos are pH-balanced, especially formulated not to strip hair of necessary oils and shine.

The more frequently you cut your hair, the faster it will grow.
Cutting does not affect the hair's growth cycle, but a trim will keep your hair looking good as it grows.

If you are on your period, you shouldn't have a perm or color your hair.
Your hair has nothing to do with your body's reproductive system.

If you have several perms or have your hair chemically straightened, eventually your hair will learn to grow that way.
Chemicals only affect the dead hair on your head, not the living hair deep inside the hair follicle.

Hair stops growing at a certain length.
Not *quite* true. Hair grows until the end of its growth cycle, which may result in very long hair for some people. You can help your hair grow longer, however, by treating it gently so it won't fall out before it has completed its full cycle.

Hair grows from the ends; that's why split ends won't grow.
Hair grows from the scalp. The ends of your hair are *old*. The longer your hair, the older the ends are (another reason older hair needs gentle treatment!).

Take a Closer Look

You'll be better able to style and understand your hair if you analyze it. You might ask a professional hair stylist for help, but you may be able to analyze your hair with your own knowhow and a mirror.

First, determine your hair's texture. Pluck a hair from a friend's head and compare your hair with hers. Is your hair thicker or narrower?

Fine hair is made up of thin, individual hairs. Fine hair is narrower and more fragile than other hair. Often natural blonde hair is fine. Girls with fine hair should never wear it pulled back. Fine hair can't stand the tension and will break easily.

Medium hair is ordinary hair, neither fine nor coarse. Brown hair is often medium.

Coarse hair is strong, almost wiry. The individual hair shafts are larger than those of fine hair. Redheads often have coarse hair.

Next, determine the curl factor of your hair. Your hair's curl is determined by the way the keratin forms in the hair cortex. The curliness of your hair can vary not only from strand to strand, but on a single hair.

Your hair's curliness can also vary throughout your life. When Angie was a baby, her hair was curly, then it straightened itself when she grew her hair into longer styles. But the last time she had her hair cut in short layers, she was surprised to find that it was curly again. Her friends thought she had permed her hair!

To best work with your hair, you should analyze your hair's oil level. The sebaceous glands, located next to the hair follicles, produce daily amounts of oil that coat the end of the hair shaft. You may have oily hair and an oily scalp, a dry scalp and dry hair (usually caused by underactive glands and/or chemical processing of your hair), or an oily scalp with dry hair (usually the result of excessive blow drying and/or chemical treatments). Make sure you use shampoos and conditioners that match the condition of your hair and scalp.

Shake Those Flakes

Dandruff is an embarrassing condition, but it's not fatal. There are two kinds of dandruff: oleosa, or oily dandruff, and sicca, or dandruff that results from a dry scalp. Dandruff can be caused by a poor diet, emotional tension, fluctuating hormones, infection, an injury to the scalp, or excessive use of hair styling aids such as hair spray or mousse.

To treat dandruff, shampoo regularly. If your scalp is normal or dry, shampoo with a dandruff shampoo once a week. If your scalp is oily, shampoo several times a week. For severe dandruff, use a tar shampoo. These loosen the dead skin on the scalp and wash it away. For lighter cases of dandruff, an ordinary dandruff shampoo such as Head 'N Shoulders will work well.

After your hair dries, brush and comb your hair carefully and thoroughly. Use a brush of soft, natural bristles, and never dig the bristles into your scalp.

Use hair products wisely. Be aware that curlers, blow dryers, and too much hair spray may damage your hair and aggravate dandruff.

Daily Habits for Lovely Locks

Everyday hair care shouldn't be a hassle. If you'll remember a few basic principles, you can develop healthy hair habits.

First, never forget that longer hair is older hair. Brush long hair gently, never pull it sharply, and never tie your hair back too tightly. Vary your hairstyles. If you wear a ponytail one day, let your hair hang free the next.

Hair is weaker when it is wet. When you get out of the shower or after you've shampooed, gently towel dry your hair. Never use a brush on wet hair; use a wide-tooth plastic comb and gently pull it through your wet hair. Start combing at the back of your head and work toward the front, handling one section at a time and detangling gently.

After you've gently worked the tangles out of your hair, let it air dry as much as possible before blow drying. Stall the blow dryer by using the time to put on your makeup, shave your legs, or pick out your clothes.

When blow drying, bend forward from the waist and hang your head down. Never hold the dryer closer than six inches to your scalp, and keep the hot air moving over the hair. Remember, heat is your hair's enemy!

When hair is nearly dry, stand up and flip your hair back. If you want smooth curls or waves, wrap a section of hair around your brush in the direction you want the curl to go. Direct the heat of the dryer over and under the wrapped hair, then let it cool for a moment before unwrapping the hair from the brush. Blow dry your bangs and other "thin hair" areas first, so they won't dry straight or frizzy.

If you have wavy hair and want to wear it straight, blow dry your hair until it is about 60 percent dry. Then use a round brush and continue drying while rolling the hair first in one direction, then the other. Unwrap your hair from the brush and alternate directions every fifteen seconds.

For perms or curly hair, use a diffuser on your dryer. The diffuser, which allows heat and air to dry the hair without blowing it "straight," slips onto the end of a blow dryer. To achieve a textured tousled look, work a little styling mousse through your hair and use your hands to "crunch" your hair while slowly drying your hair with a diffuser. Bending over from the waist while drying will give your hair more volume.

When you're ready to brush your hair, make sure your brush is clean. You can keep brushes and combs clean by soaking them occasionally in warm, soapy water. Scrub your brushes gently with an old toothbrush, and dry brushes with the bristles facing down.

Brushing is an important beauty exercise that stimulates the scalp, increases circulation, distributes oils, and adds fullness and shine to your hair. But be careful. Over-brushing can cause hair to break. Be gentle with your hair!

To brush properly, don't start at the front of your forehead and brush backward—the hair at your forehead is delicate and easily broken. Instead, bend forward at the waist, start at the back neckline, and brush while working toward the front. Rip your hair back, and use the brush to smooth your hair into place.

When should you brush your hair? Today's experts say that Grandma's prescription for one hundred strokes before bedtime is really too much brushing, but bedtime isn't a bad time to brush. Give your hair a thorough brushing in the morning, in the evening before bed, and always brush carefully before shampooing to loosen dirt so it can be washed away.

When you and your hair are ready for a good night's sleep, remove everything from your hair, including pins, headbands, and stiffly sprayed curls. Your hair needs to relax at night, too!

The Right Shampoo

If you had to stand in the grocery store and choose the best shampoo, you could go a little nuts. There are millions (well, hundreds) of varieties and brands from which to choose, and there are even more if you consider those sold in beauty salons. Until the 1930s, people had it easy — cake soap was the only way to clean hair. (Can you imagine rubbing your hair down with a bar of soap?)

But you can make an informed choice about which shampoo is best for you. Buy a shampoo that fits your hair type—one for oily hair, dry hair, dandruff, or color-treated hair. There are shampoos for permed hair, and shampoos for blondes, brunettes, and redheads. By the way, don't be afraid to switch shampoos once in a while. You might find one you like better.

Do steer clear of "conditioning" shampoos that clean and condition hair at the same time. These contain lanolin, which coats the hair with oil. You'll end up with hair that's slightly gummy.

For the perfect shampoo, first wet your hair, using water as warm as possible. Next, apply a minimum amount of shampoo, about the size of a fifty-cent piece. Squeeze the shampoo into your palm first, so you can see how much you're using, rub your hands together, then apply the shampoo to your hair. Work it into your hair and scalp, starting on the top of your head and working down the length of your hair. Be firm, but not rough. Concentrate your efforts around the hairline and neckline.

Rinsing is very important. To rinse long hair, lift small sections under the running water and work your way up. If you're in the shower, you should bend forward and let the water hit your back neckline, then stand up and let the shower rinse your front hairline. To assure a complete rinse, keep a plastic squirt bottle filled with a mix of one-half cup apple cider vinegar and one-half cup water in the shower. Squirt it through your hair, and stand under the running water for another rinse. The apple cider vinegar mix will not only leave your hair clean, but it brings out the highlights in your hair.

After shampooing, your hair needs a conditioner. All hair needs conditioning, but some hair needs it more than others. The sun, wind, chlorine, blow drying, hot curlers, curling irons, mousses, gels with alcohol-all these dry the hair. *Everyone* needs hair conditioner.

Conditioners don't penetrate the hair, they coat it and fill in the cracks around the cuticle to help the hair retain moisture. To apply conditioner, mix a small amount (about the size of a quarter) in a cup of hot water, and pour the mixture on your hair, beginning at two inches from the scalp and down. Work the mixture down to the ends, where hair is the driest. You may find it helpful to use a wide-tooth comb to distribute the mixture evenly. Leave the conditioner on for at least a minute, rinse with warm water, then finish with a cold-water rinse. The cold water shrinks the cuticles of the hair shaft, causing them to lie flat.

Not all conditioners are designed to be used in the shower. Some are "deep conditioning treatments" for severely damaged hair. These conditioners should be used every two to four weeks.

If you'd like to try a simple home treatment for damaged hair, hair stylist Louis Gignac suggests that you warm 1/4 cup pure olive oil on the stove. With a cotton ball, apply the oil lightly to the ends of your hair and any damaged spots. Comb the oil through the hair with a wide-tooth comb, then wrap your head in a sheet of aluminum foil and sit in the sun or under a hair dryer for fifteen minutes. Unwrap your head and shampoo your hair twice. If the hair is still oily, mix half a cup of apple cider vinegar with half a cup of water and rinse. This treatment is safe for all hair.[2]

To add natural shine to your hair, squeeze and strain the juice of half a lemon into one cup of cold water. Stir. Pour onto your hair and leave on three minutes, then rinse with cold water. If you'd prefer to use a packaged product to encourage hair shine, you might try Jose Eber's Luminizing Enhancing Mist, L'Oreal's Colorvive Instant Shine Booster, or Alberto's FrizzSolver and Shine Enhancer. Be sure to read the label carefully, because these products must be used properly and sparingly. Too much will only weigh your hair down.

No time to shampoo? Sprinkle baby powder or baking soda through your hair and brush thoroughly.

Want a special lift on a hot day? Dab cologne or perfume around your hairline. The alcohol in the perfume will not only remove excess oil, but it's refreshing and smells good, too.

Tools for Mane-tenance

After your hair is washed, dried, and brushed, how do you get it into shape? If you haven't used your blow dryer as a styling aid, you will probably reach now for a hairstyling tool.

If you don't have the patience for a curling iron, *heated rollers* are the quickest tools to put curl into your hair. Leave hot rollers in for between five and fifteen minutes, depending on how much curl you want, then brush your hair thoroughly. Always unwind rollers carefully; don't just yank them out.

Velcro™ rollers are convenient because they don't require clips or pins to hold them in place. If your hair is still damp, roll it on

11

Velcro™ rollers and continue blow drying for a firm curl. (To perk up dry, flat hair, roll it up on Velcro™ rollers, spray lightly with hair spray, allow the spray to dry, and then unwind rollers. Your hair will be full again.)

Curling irons are quick but tricky to use. When wrapping your hair in a curling iron, make sure all the ends of the hair are inside the iron before curling. Some curling irons feature bristles like a brush, and these are often easier to use because they grip hair and hold it in place.

Crimping and waving irons are fun and create more unusual hairstyles. *Straightening irons* will press the curl out of hair, but also reduce volume.

Hair benders are soft, pliable rods used on damp hair to give a loose curl. They work well on long hair.

Flat irons can straighten and smooth frizzy hair, but if you turn your wrist, you could put a curl in your hair. That's fine—if it's what you meant to do.

Some of the best hair styling aids come in a bottle. *Styling gel or paste* is used for greater hold and control. Gels work well when blow drying or sculpting the hair for a "slicked back" look. Gel also helps accentuate spiked or curly textures in hair.

Hair spray does more than hold hair in a finished style. You can use hair spray to encourage curls as you wrap hair around rollers, while your hair is in rollers, and before you brush freshly set curls out. Hair spray comes in many different strengths, so select one that suits the amount of hold your style needs.

Styling lotions can protect hair from the heat of blow dryers and heated rollers. Styling lotions come in strong, "designing spray" formulas that allow you to style your hair in any form you can imagine. Styling lotions are great for fine hair because they are not as heavy as gels and won't flatten hair.

Chemical Solutions

The urge to perm comes and goes in our culture. When Angie was a teenager, long, straight hair was in style, and those who had naturally curly hair were reduced to ironing it on their moms' ironing boards or rolling it on orange juice cans to get the kinks out!

As silly as it seems, that old routine may be healthier for hair than the current trend to perm. When you perm your hair, strong chemicals break the molecular chains of the cortex of your hair and mold the hair to the shape on the curling rod. In order for the hair to keep its new curly shape, the broken molecular chains must be reformed, so a neutralizing solution is applied at exactly the right moment. This neutralizer shrinks and hardens the cortex layer of hair.

A *body wave* is done by the exact same process, but the curlers, or rods, are larger than those used for a curly perm. A body wave is a perm that adds form and volume instead of oodles of curls.

The advantages to a perm are obvious—you can shampoo your hair, towel it dry, shake your head, and that's it. Permed hair is wash-and-wear, and a good perm lasts three months before the new growth of straight hair becomes noticeable. (Chemically curled hair is exactly what its name says: *permanent*. The curl may loosen, but it is curled forever.)

Chemical *straightening* does exactly the opposite of a permanent. Curly hair is saturated with a permanent solution, combed straight, and neutralized. The more often your hair is straightened, the dryer it becomes. There is a mild straightening solution that takes out only 79 percent of the curl, but strong solutions will leave your hair absolutely straight.

A perm *may* be ideal for you and your lifestyle ... and it may not. Never have a chemical solution applied on a whim, but think the decision through carefully.

Color-Perfect!

Before you attempt to change your natural hair color, ask yourself why you want a different color. You're too young to worry about covering gray hair, so if you want to change your hair color so you'll look like a friend or a movie star, you may be forgetting that you are a unique person. Your hair is probably perfect for your skin tone and your eye color. And keep in mind, the farther away the new color is from your natural color, the more damaged your hair will be in the color process.

Today there are all kinds of color treatments that can give your hair a quick lift. Some of these can be done at home, others should be done in a salon. Some hair color treatments are permanent, others are temporary and wash out with shampoo. Read every label carefully before you attempt to do anything, and talk to your parents before doing anything drastic to your hair.

Laura suggests trying a *semi-permanent* color before making a commitment to a permanent color change. Semi-permanent colors are applied like shampoo and left on for about twenty minutes. These colors will fade gradually with each shampoo and will not leave a growth line in your hair. Semi-permanent colors cannot be used, however, to *lighten* hair. They can darken, redden, brighten, and add shine, but they cannot lighten hair because they do not contain bleaching agents.

Other temporary colors come in the form of colored rinses, colored mousse, and colored gels. These are a fun way to experiment, but you should not use a bright gel or mousse on bleached or very light hair. They can stain and are difficult to remove.

Highlights are a great alternative to an overall dye job. A coloring agent is applied to small sections of hair pulled through a rubber cap or wrapped in individual pieces of foil. Highlighting gives hair a brighter, sun-lightened effect. Choose a tint only one or two shades lighter than your own color.

Highlighting brightens drab blonde or red hair color and gives beautiful auburn highlights to dark brown hair. If you really want professional results, have it done in a salon every two or three months.

Lowlights are achieved through the same process as highlights, but the tints are one or two shades *darker* than your own color. This is the best way to make your color slightly darker, to cut down bright red shades, or to allow previously bleached hair to grow out less noticeably.

Before doing anything to your hair, be sure you know what you are doing. Many "home jobs" can look tacky or obvious, and the point of hair coloring is to look as *natural as possible*. You don't want people noticing your beautiful blonde streaks; you want them to notice the beautiful *you*. If you are determined to change your hair color, Laura suggests that you have it done professionally, at least for the first few times. While your hair is being colored, watch carefully and ask questions so that in the future you might be able to do it the same at home. (Professional beauty supply stores can also give you a wealth of information and advice.)

Finding the Perfect Hairstyle for You

"Oh. That hairstyle would be darling on you!" Well, maybe it would, and maybe it wouldn't. Practically any hairstyle can be adapted to be worn by any girl, but some styles will work better for you than others. You should always consider all of the following before allowing the stylist to give you a new haircut:

1. *Your face/body shape:* Forget about all those complicated diagrams. Just pull your hair back and look in the mirror. Now take a bar of soap, close one eye, and "draw" around your face's reflection in the mirror. Now stand back and evaluate. Is your face round, oval, or long?

Now that you have an idea of your facial shape, remember that you are more than a face. You also should consider your neck length, your torso, and your height when considering a hairstyle.

Women with large frames should avoid super-short haircuts; they need hair to provide balance. Small women should avoid super-long hair because long hair tends to bury its owners. Ask your stylist what he or she recommends for your face and body shape. Or go to the Internet and search for hairstyles for your face shape—you'll find zillions of photos, so print out your faves and take them to your hairdresser.

A few tips: If your ears stick out, by all means, cover them with hair. Don't opt for a super short cut. If your nose is large and prominent, avoid a center part or straight, heavy bangs. If you are big-boned, you may want to find a style with volume for balance. If you have wide shoulders, shoulder-length hair will narrow your look. Girls with low foreheads should avoid bangs, and girls with wide foreheads may look best with bangs.

2.   *Your hair type:* Is your hair naturally curly, frizzy, or straight? Layered styles encourage curl; long, blunt cuts pull curl out. Straight-as-a-board hair won't work well in wavy or curly dos unless you want to perm or spend twenty minutes every morning with a curling iron. Frizzy hair will never be sleek or straight without a chemical treatment, but a curling iron will take the frizzies out if you opt for a more controlled style.

3.   *Your hair/scalp type:* Is your hair/scalp combo dry, oily, or a combination of the two? If your hair is oily and you'll be shampooing every day, consider a wash-and-wear cut and style.

4.   *Your hair's body:* Is your hair naturally thick, fine, or

15

normal? Fine hair shouldn't be all one length. Layers will make fine hair look thicker, and a perm can add volume.

For thick hair, a layered cut works best. Your stylist can adjust the layers to "fit" your facial shape, and a good cut is crucial. Blunt cuts do not work well on thick hair unless you want to look like Cleopatra.

Do not let a stylist take thinning shears to thick hair. If your hair is too thick for a particular style, you'd be better off to have your hair layered than to have it thinned. Thinning shears, which randomly cut hairs, can cause hair to frizz.

The Long and Short of It!

Most girls adore long hair, and they overlook some of the wonderful things shorter hair can do to enhance beauty.

"Short" hair, cut above chin length, is charming, bouncy, and cute. Short hair needs more upkeep and more frequent cuts to keep it sharp and in shape, and short hair is often less versatile than longer hair. But short hair is great if you are athletic. Princess Diana, Katie Couric, and Laura have short hair and love it!

"Medium" hair, cut above the shoulders, is versatile. You can pull medium length hair up, wear it down, fluff it out, or smooth it back. There are a thousand medium length hairstyles, and your stylist can help you discover the best one for you.

"Long" hair that is at least shoulder length, needs lots of tender loving care. Long hair is not as versatile as medium hair, but it can be braided and pulled back. Long hair should be kept trimmed and conditioned regularly. If you choose to wear long hair, don't fall into the trap of just letting it grow without rhyme or reason. Keep your long hair styled, in good condition, and dress it up for special occasions!

The Key to Success

The key to a good-looking hairstyle is a great hair cut. Never, ever walk into a salon and accept an appointment with any available hair stylist unless you're willing to spend the next six months or so growing out what could be a mistake. If you want a really good cut, go on a scouting expedition first. Find a friend whose hair you like or sit in the mall until you see someone with a nice style and cut. Look for non-fussy hair that swings with bounce and shine. Then, don't be shy. Ask this lucky girl who cuts her hair.

Once you have the name of a stylist and salon, call the salon and ask if you can come in for a free consultation. Any salon that's good will agree. Show up for your appointment on time, and be prepared to make a little speech like this:

"Hello, I'm (your name) and I'm looking for a new hairstyle. I only have about (how many?) minutes a day to spend on my hair, and I like (or don't like) to spend a lot of time on it. I want a look that's (classy, sporty, sophisticated, smooth, bouncy, funky, contemporary—choose one or come up with your own adjectives). I want to emphasize my good features and downplay my weak ones."

Be sure to tell the stylist if you apply chemicals to your hair or regularly use any hair coloring products, perms, straighteners, etc. Let the stylist know what tools (blow dryer, hot curlers, flat iron, gel, paste, bobby pins) you like to use in styling your hair, and which you don't. If you have a photograph of a style you like, show it to the stylist, but don't expect to enter *any* salon and come out looking exactly like the picture. After you've done these things, smile sweetly and ask: "So . . . what would you suggest?"

If the stylist is good, he or she will listen to you carefully and answer your questions without making you feel stupid. While you're having your consultation, take a careful look around. Who are the clientele? Are there other teenagers in the salon, or is the place full of older ladies in pin curls? What type of products are for sale? What are the other stylists doing — using lots of hair spray, teasing (uh-oh!), using hot rollers?

Don't be afraid to ask about prices and how long you will typically have to wait to get an appointment (the really good stylists are often booked up weeks in advance). As you leave, ask the receptionist, "How easy is it to get in with so-and-so if I need an appointment in a week?"

If all the signs are favorable, make an appointment to have your hair cut and styled. If you don't like what you see at the salon, you're free to walk out with a smile and try another place.

Before the Snipping Starts

Before you and the stylist take the first step toward a new hair cut, remember that a good haircut should be versatile. Settle on a style that allows you to wear your hair in at least two different looks, casual and dressy. Some styles can be worn several different ways.

Your stylist should look at your hair when it is dry and cut it when it is wet. If someone attempts to cut your hair while it is dry, jump out of the chair and run. (This, of course, doesn't pertain to those last-minute touch up snips after your hair has been cut and blown dry.)

When it is time for your haircut, the stylist will drape an apron around your neck. Your hair should be wet, and he should carefully comb it through, then pick up his scissors. A good stylist will pick up a section of hair, hold the scissors up, look at you in the mirror, and say, "This is where I'm planning to cut. Right?" Make sure that first cut is where you thought it would be. Hair will shorten as it dries, so it's better to have your hair too long than too short.

When the haircut is finished, give your new cut the shakeout test You should be able to hang your head down, give it a shake, then flip it up. Does your hair fall naturally back into shape? If it does, you've had a good cut.

Bill Baker, a photographer and hair stylist, encourages teenagers to talk freely to their stylists. "Teenagers often don't know what they want, but they know what they don't want," he says. "They come in and give all sorts of restrictions to the stylist, and often they are unrealistic. Each person's hair will only do certain things. A lot of girls bring in a picture and want to look just like the picture, but they haven't yet learned what their hair will do."

Baker also encourages girls to be unique. "A lot of girls follow the crowd. That baffles me. Their hair isn't in style; you won't find a hairdo like theirs in a single fashion magazine. But girls haven't yet discovered the advantage in being unique. They just want to do what their friends are doing."

Special Occasion Dos

If you're planning to have your hair done at the salon for a special occasion, don't wait until the big day to have your hair styled. Make an appointment the week before and have a "test run" of your hairdo. "A lot of girls come in to have their hair done for prom or whatever," says Baker, "and they'll try anything—braids, twists, whatever. They want to be different, but when they see the result, it's too different, so they freak out and leave in tears. You should always try out a new hairstyle before the big occasion."

So whatever condition your hair is in, make the most of it. Our hair was intended to be our crowning glory, so enjoy it.

2
THE SKIN YOU'RE IN

Wanakee, a well-known model, has good advice for girls who want the best for their skin:

> I believe that beauty should be plain and practical. I love the simplicity of a bar of glycerin soap and a Buf Puf® followed by a facial moisturizer. I generally stay away from the expensive specialty creams and exotic cosmetic remedies. A good cleansing astringent and a cotton ball can work wonders on trouble spots, such as blemishes on the back and shoulders, as well as the forehead.

Of all the vital organs in our bodies, we probably take our skin most for granted. You know you can't live without a heart or lungs or kidneys, but did you ever stop to think about the importance of your skin?

You live in a God-designed suit of skin that would cover twenty-one square feet if stretched out flat. Your skin cools you in summer, warms you in winter, throws off body waste, and fights attacking organisms that try to enter your body. Skin is truly a miracle, but we scratch it, scrub it, scribble it, burn it, pinch it, bruise it, and generally abuse it. Still our skin keeps doing its job.

The top layer of your skin, the *stratum corneum,* is a protective armor against heat, sun, and external injuries. It varies in thickness from the thick pad of calluses at your heels to the delicate lining of your eyelids.

Below the top layer of skin is the *stratum lucidum*, a clear layer. Under that is a granular layer, then the *stratum germinativum*, a prickle cell layer. Finally, under all these layers of protection with hard-to-pronounce names is the *basal cell layer*, where skin cells are formed. Skin cells gravitate upward from the basal cell layer and are cast off regularly, every twenty-five days or so. This process is called keratinization, and through this process your skin is constantly renewing itself.

Your skin layers contain sebaceous glands (just like those in the scalp) that manufacture oil to lubricate your skin and hair. The skin also contains sweat glands, hair follicles, blood and lymph vessels, nerve-ending cells, muscles, and fat. In fact, one square inch of skin contains: 78 nerves

- 650 sweat glands
- 10 or 20 blood vessels
- 78 sensors for heat 13 sensors for cold
- 1,300 nerve endings to record pain 19,500 sensory cells at the end of nerve fibers 160-165 pressure (touch) sensors
- 95-100 oil-producing sebaceous glands
- 65 hairs and muscles
- 19,000,000 cells!

The Essential Lube Job

Now that we've had our biology lesson about skin, you'll understand that the sebaceous glands of your skin manufacture *sebum*, a natural body lubricant. When the sebaceous glands are too active, acne results, and over 80 percent of teenagers will suffer at some point from some form of acne and its resulting bumps, pimples, and blackheads. If you have ever found yourself wishing that your oil glands would take a holiday, you're not alone!

Why do our sebaceous glands go out of control? Hormones. When your hormones rev up in puberty and begin changing your body, the sebaceous glands are stimulated to secrete extra amounts of sebum on the surface of the skin. This extra oil mixes with discarded skin scales from the follicle walls and bacteria, and soon you have a plugged up pore. The result is whiteheads *(milia)* or blackheads *(comedones)*. Blackheads are plugged pores where the oil has darkened through exposure to the air. Whiteheads result from follicles that have closed off.

If the excess sebum has no exit from the under-layers of the skin, it stays below the surface in the follicle and causes a red, raised bump. White corpuscles race to fight the infection that occurs and the result is a nasty, pus-filled pimple.

But don't feel like the Lone Ranger when you get a pimple. Most girls (adults, too) have acne outbreaks at the beginning of each menstrual period, when estrogen hormone production goes down and causes a hormone imbalance. Other causes of acne are stress, too many fats in the diet, oily skin inherited from a parent, infections in the body, and poor personal hygiene.

The A-Word

Four out of five teenagers have acne, and we know some adults fail to take the condition seriously. "Just relax and get more sleep," someone may tell you. Or "It's because you're eating chocolate, you know. Just wait and you'll grow out of it."

Fortunately, good personal hygiene can do a lot to relieve acne. You should keep your skin dry and toned without making it red and sore. Think about your personal habits — do you often lean your chin or your cheek on your hand? Our hands carry zillions of germs, and if you constantly have your hands on your face, you're transferring germs to a sticky, oily surface that will trap those nasty bacteria like Velcro™.

Do you wear a tight sweatband on your forehead? Do you often pick at your skin? Do you hold a musical instrument against your face? Do you work around grease that spatters on your skin? Do you often use skin care products or sun screens with oil or lanolin? If so, you may be aggravating your acne.

Acne varies in severity from occasional mild outbreaks to deep boils over the face, neck, and back. If your acne is severe, you should consult a physician or dermatologist. If your acne is mild, there are several things you can do at home to help your skin.

Zit-zappers

First, analyze your skin. To determine if your skin is oily or dry, rub a piece of a brown paper bag over your face when you first get up in the morning. If the paper turns dark, you have oily skin. If there is only a slight stain, your skin is normal. If there is no stain, your skin is dry.

Whatever your skin type, keep your skin clean. It is vital to remove the oil and grease from the skin at least twice a day. Remember, bacteria breeds in oil, and this may mean washing your face several times a day, followed by careful rinsing and gentle drying. Use an antiseptic soap that kills bacteria and germs.

Depending upon the severity of your acne, you may wish to use an abrasive product such as Aapri Apricot Facial Scrub, which contains tiny grains of sand that loosen blackheads and the upper layer of the corneum. Whenever you're using a facial scrub, pretend you are wearing a pair of large sunglasses. Do not do any scrubbing in the areas that would be covered by the imaginary lenses. The gentle skin around your eyes can't handle rough treatment.

If you develop a pus-filled bump, or lesion, it must be dried out. You can use a medicated lotion that contains sulfur, salicylic acid, resorcinol, or benzoyl peroxide. If areas of your face are red and swollen, treat those areas with compresses of boric acid and Burow's solution. Use cosmetics with care, and avoid greasy products, foundations, or creams.

If your skin is very oily, use an astringent several times a week. Look for astringents without skin-drying alcohol. The best astringents contain acetone or witch hazel.

To fight acne, you should also keep your hair and scalp clean. Avoid greasy or sticky hair products or conditioners with lanolin.

Give oily skin a fighting chance by keeping your hands off your face. Squeezing pimples can spread infection.

You may find that your acne is helped tremendously if you change your diet. Zinc supplements have been known to clear up problem acne, but you should use them only under a doctor's supervision. Maureen Salaman, a nutritionist, found that fifty milligrams of elemental zinc three times a day with meals worked "miracles" with acne patients. You can get your zinc naturally by eating herring, wheat germ, sesame seeds, liver, soybeans, sunflower seeds, egg yolks, and lamb.

Ask the Doctor

If you choose to see a doctor for acne problems, he or she may prescribe antibiotics to help your condition. Drugs such as tetracycline, erythromycin, and vibramycin work to suppress the formation of unsaturated fatty acids which produce acne lesions, but these drugs are expensive and have been known to produce side effects of nausea, diarrhea, and yeast infections. (If you are taking antibiotics, be sure to eat at least eight ounces of fat-free yogurt daily to prevent the decrease of "helpful" bacteria in the intestines which antibiotics often destroy.) Some antibiotics are available as a lotion that can be applied directly to the skin.

Dermatologists also offer treatments to help skin that has been scarred by past bouts of acne. *Dermabrasion* is the process in which the facial skin is frozen, then a motor-driven brush gently runs over the face, "sanding" away the excessive scar tissue. The face will form a protective crust that lasts about a week, and the underlying skin will be red for several weeks.

Peeling often helps shallow acne pits. A mild acid solution is applied to the skin, and the top layer peels off in seven to ten days.

Chemotherapy is used to treat deeper scarring. Trichloroacetic acid is used on the skin, and the peeling persists for two to three weeks.

As you can see, these acne treatments are extreme, but for people with severe acne they provide wonderful relief. If yours is moderate to mild acne, do your best to keep your skin healthy and clear through proper diet, hygiene, and care.

A Program for Care of Normal Skin

If your skin is normal, wash your face every night with your favorite water-soluble soap. Think *gentle*. Avoid bar soaps, especially if your skin feels tight after washing with them. Your soap should leave your skin feeling soft, not greasy, and it should also remove eye makeup.

Be sure to wash with warm (not hot!) water. Two or three times a week, substitute a scrub (like Aapri Apricot Gentle Facial Scrub) for your usual cleanser or massage a generous portion of baking soda over your skin. Baking soda is gentle, plus it's an anti-inflammatory agent that doesn't inflame your skin as some scrubs or other harsh cleansers can.

If your skin feels tight even after using a gentle soap, use an oil-free moisturizer on your cheeks. Don't moisturize your nose, chin, or forehead. This "T-zone" has enough oil glands to keep your skin smooth.

Whenever you have blemishes, pimples, or clogged pores, massage a generous portion of baking soda over the blemished area, then rinse completely. Twice a day, soak a cotton ball in 3 percent hydrogen peroxide and apply the solution to the infected areas or areas of your face that tend to break out. Hydrogen peroxide is gentle, inexpensive, and it disinfects your skin. With consistent use, it will actually lighten blackheads. Be careful, though, about using hydrogen peroxide around your hairline and eyebrows. It will also lighten your hair!

Every morning, cleanse your face with soap and warm water. If you're going to spend much time outdoors, spread small dabs of low-oil sunscreen on your face, and let the sunscreen dry before you apply your makeup.

A Program for Oily Skin

If your skin is oily, wash your face thoroughly every night with warm water and a soap such as Neutrogena for Oily Skin or Basis. Rinse carefully, first with five handfuls of warm water, then with three handfuls of cool water. Dry your face with a fluffy towel, then use a cotton ball to apply an astringent such as Ten-O-Six or witch hazel.

Every morning, cleanse your face with your bar soap as you did at night. Apply astringent with a clean cotton ball. Two or three times a week you may consider using a scrub such as Buf Puf Cleansing Pads, Seven Day Scrub Cream (Clinique), or Clean and Clear Cleansing Bar (Revlon).

Use only oil-free makeup such as Clinique's Pore Minimizer Makeup or Maybelline's oil-free makeups such as Shine Free. If you're in doubt about a makeup, read the label. Avoid products that contain mineral oil and/or lanolin.

Oily skin can vary from season to season. You may find that your skin is oilier in summer than winter, so don't scrub skin that is too dry. Remember, even oily skin deserves gentle care. You only have one face.

A Program for Dry Skin Care

If your skin is dry, cleanse your face every night with a gentle cleaner such as Olay Beauty Cleanser or Estee Lauder's Instant Action Rinse-off Cleanser. Rinse very well, splashing ten to fifteen handfuls of warm water on your face. Dry your face gently with an absorbent towel. Pat on a nighttime moisturizer.

Each morning, cleanse your face as you did at night. Apply a moisturizing astringent such as Clinique's Alcohol-free Clarifier or Revlon's Moon Drops Moisturizing Skin Toner for dry skin, and allow your face to dry. After toning, use a lightweight, deep-penetrating water-based moisturizer. Apply makeup. If your skin is very dry, concentrate on cream-based makeups, lipsticks, and blushes. Avoid "frosted" cosmetics because they contain minerals that soak up your skin's natural oils.

Avoid oily makeup in the oily "T" zone, and use a moisturizer in the dry areas. If your skin is dry and flakes or chaps easily, wash with a gentle, creamy soap and use gentle-formula cosmetics.

Remember, dry skin is aggravated by dehydration so you'll need to drink lots of water. Dehydration increases if you're often in central heating, live in an extremely hot or cold climate, or if you're traveling in an airplane. Caffeine, sun exposure, and certain prescribed medicines also cause your body to lose water, so remember to drink lots of H2O.

Eating for Beautiful Skin

Whatever your skin type, you can help your skin by eating green and yellow veggies, fruits, eggs, milk, butter, and fruit juices. Don't forget to drink lots of water every day, and get eight hours of sleep every night. Skin cells do most of their growing when your body is at rest. Why do you think they call it "beauty sleep"?

Bathing—A Beauty Basic

Archaeologists have found bathtubs in private homes from 3000 B.C., and we know the ancient Romans built immense public baths, but there was a time in medieval human history when bathing was considered eccentric. A lot of grimy, stinky people walked around beneath layers of gorgeous clothes. Their uncleanness contributed to plagues, skin sores, and disease.

The simple act of bathing (or showering, of course) kills germs and viruses by the zillions. Soap and water loosen the grime and dirt on our skin where bacteria and viruses breed. When you rinse yourself, all those dead and dying germs are washed down the drain.

You may not realize it, but in the course of a typical day your skin becomes coated with an invisible layer of whatever is in the air dust, smog, insecticide sprays, poisons, and other irritants. The warm water of a bath or shower opens your pores, dilates the blood vessels, and relaxes your body tissues. That's why you feel better when you're squeaky clean.

A good, old-fashioned tub bath has other psychological benefits, too. A bath relaxes you and helps you sleep. Plus, while you're soaking in the tub, you have the opportunity to soften and scrub your tough heels, elbows, and toes with a pumice stone. Bath oils are good for temporarily lubricating your skin, and bath salts and bubble baths can be fun. (Just don't use too much bath products have been known to cause kidney infections.)

Bathing for Beginners (Pretend That's You)

Though you've been bathing for years, let's pretend you've been scooped up out of a deep jungle somewhere and you're about to be introduced to a bathtub or shower. First, make sure your water is warm, not hot. Very hot or very cold water can damage the skin and reduce the natural oils that keep your skin supple.

Now ease yourself into the water. Ahh, that feels great. Now grab your soap and start lathering up, but remember to work from the top down. Pay special attention to the creased areas of your body where bacteria hide and breed your armpits, your private areas, between your toes. After you're lathered up, use a soapy washcloth or a bath sponge to wipe grime and invisible bacteria off and away from your skin.

After you've wiped yourself clean, reach for a long-handled brush and give your back a good scrub. You'll spare your back an entire crop of blackheads and blemishes with regular cleansing. After a good rinse with warm water, you're ready to head into a thick, absorbent, clean bath towel. There. Don't you feel better?

Hair Today, Gone Tomorrow!

While we're on the subject of skin, let's consider the thousands of hairs that grow all over your body. We live in a culture that promotes the sleek, smooth look, so what's the best way to smooth out your legs and underarms?

Shaving is probably the easiest, quickest, and most economical way to remove unwanted hair on your legs and underarms. The process is very simple.

1.   Use lots of water. Shaving is best accomplished after a long soak in the tub or just after you've come out of a warm

shower.

2.   Use shaving cream or a product like Soft Shave to soften up the hairs on your legs. Make sure your legs are wet, then apply shaving cream. Shave carefully, in short strokes, and rinse your razor often. Clean blades shave more evenly, and you won't have to press on the razor.

3.   Be sure your razor is sharp. If you have to repeat a stroke to pick up hair the razor missed on the first pass, it's time to replace your razor. Never use a clogged or rusted razor.

4.   After your shave, rinse your legs with warm water. Apply a soothing, alcohol-free lotion, and you're done. Allow your razor to air dry, and never wipe the blades with a towel or tissue.

Shaving tips: During the summer months, shave the night before your day at the beach or pool to avoid irritation from the sun, salt, or chlorine. Never shave over a sunburn. If you develop itchy red bumps the day after shaving, try shaving in the opposite direction the next time you shave. Finally, a word of warning— never shave any part of your face!

Waxing. Shaving cuts hair at the skin level, but waxing removes hair from below the skin surface so the hair takes longer to grow back. If you decide to wax your legs, first arrange to have it professionally done to see if waxing is really a good option for you. If it is, the next time you can purchase a waxing kit at the drugstore or beauty supply shop and follow the directions carefully.

If you're curious about what's involved, the waxing procedure is this: First you wash your skin with an antiseptic soap, then you apply the wax over your skin in the direction of hair growth. A strip of cloth is placed over the wax, and as the wax dries, it fastens to the cloth. When the wax is dried, you rip the cloth, the wax, and your hair away. Ouch!

Depilatories. Chemical depilatories like Nair are less painful than waxing and last from six to eight weeks. But before you cover your legs with the chemicals, first test a small area of skin to make sure you don't have an allergic reaction. Laura once had a bad experience with a depilatory, so she warns that you must wait twenty-four hours after you have tested your skin. After twenty-four hours, if your skin has suffered no ill effects, you can proceed. Apply the mixture as directed on the package, wait the allotted time, then wash away the solution with soap and water.

Electrolysis is an expensive, permanent method of hair removal that must be performed by a professional. The electrologist gently inserts a small platinum needle into each hair follicle until it reaches the papilla at the base. Then an electric current is turned on and the hair bulb is zapped. As a result, the hair bulb coagulates. It's dead. The hair is then removed from the dead follicle with tweezers, and no hair will grow from that hair bulb again. Of course, if you were to have your legs done with electrolysis, it would take several sessions to cover each and every hair follicle. Most people choose electrolysis for smaller jobs, like eyebrows or other facial hair.

Laura warns that electrolysis can be painful, and if not properly done, scarring may result. Electrolysis should be performed only by professionals.

Bearded Lady?

We don't know why facial hair should be embarrassing, because if s only natural that if you have dark brown or black hair you also have dark hair on your face. Some girls are mortified to think they have a moustache. You don't have to suffer embarrassment, though, because there are two simple things you can do.

You can choose to bleach the dark hair above your lip. There are several creams available at your drug store that will lighten facial hair so that it is hardly noticeable (Jolen Creme Bleach is excellent).

Be forewarned — a bleach may work beautifully for you, but often bleach turns facial hair yellow. Is yellow facial hair better than dark? You may wish to use a chemical depilatory especially designed for facial hair, and simply wash that hair away. Don't use any chemical, however, unless it is specifically formulated for facial hair. A depilatory for your legs may be too strong for your face. As with any chemical, do a test first and wait twenty-four hours before proceeding.

If you bleach your facial hair, you won't have to worry about the regrowth of dark hairs. But no matter which method you choose, you'll have to repeat the treatment once every week or two, but you can do it in the privacy of your room.

The Fragrance That Flatters

Once you're out of the tub and clean, perfume can help you carry a fresh feeling with you through the day. Perfume in its truest form (the expensive stuff) is 70-85 percent alcohol and 15-30 percent essence — fixatives and pure oils. Toilet water is mid-way between perfume and cologne, which contains up to 95 percent alcohol and 5 percent essence.

Buy (or request) your first good perfume carefully. We are of the opinion that it's better to have one or two perfumes in several formulas (toilet water, powder, body lotion) than bottles of five or six different scents. The sense of smell is very strong, and we often associate a certain scent with a particular memory of a person, place, or time. Why not choose a fragrance that reflects your personality for your own "signature scent"? Whenever that certain guy smells it, he'll think of you!

If you're shopping for a scent to call your own, don't test more than two or three fragrances at a time. Remember, you can't judge a scent solely on how it smells in the bottle or how it smells on your friend. You have to let the oils react with your own skin's chemistry, and you shouldn't have more than two or three scents mixed up on your wrist.

Once you've found a fragrance that you're wild about, build your fragrance wardrobe and apply it carefully as you get dressed in the morning. You might apply a deodorant/antiperspirant in your scent, then powder your skin in your scent's body powder. (Fill a small container with a little body powder and a powder puff and toss it into your purse for an after-gym or midday freshen up!) Rub a little scented lotion onto your knees and elbows, then apply your toilet water, perfume, or cologne to your pulse points—your wrists, at the base of your neck, behind your ears. You may find it helpful to spread a thin layer of petroleum jelly on these areas before you apply fragrance. Some say the jelly helps fragrance last longer.

You'll probably notice that after a while you can no longer smell your fragrance. That's a result of nose fatigue. Our noses have the ability to "block out" scents after a certain period of time, and if you are able to smell your scent thirty minutes after you've applied fragrance, you've overdone it. If you've over-applied your favorite fragrance, saturate a cotton ball with rubbing alcohol and dab it on the skin where you applied the perfume. The alcohol will cut the scent without altering it.

When purchasing your favorite fragrance, don't buy the gallon-sized bottle. Fragrances have a relatively short shelf life, and if your bottle is too big or if you stock up on too many fragrances, you won't be able to use them all before they turn to alcohol. Perfumes have a shelf life of twelve to fourteen months; colognes are at their best only for six months.

For an especially refreshing treat, store your fragrances in the fridge. Don't allow them to sit in sunlight, and don't transfer your perfumes to plastic bottles. The chemical reaction between the plastic and the perfume's oils will alter the balance of ingredients.

Years ago the Avon slogan was "Whatever you wear, wear fragrance!" You should. There are hundreds of wonderful perfumes and colognes on the market, in every price range. Find one that expresses your innermost self, and wear it proudly.

To Tan or Not to Tan ...

The song says ol' Mister Sun has nothing to do but roll around heaven all day, but the sun is doing a lot more than that. He's frying people. Until seventy years ago, a lily-white or peaches-and-cream complexion was revered among women. Genteel ladies wore gloves and wide hats and carried parasols to keep Mister Sun away. But in the 1920s, when Coco Chanel came back from her sunny vacation, women decided that tan was in. A tan was a sign of beauty and robust health, and it also implied that its wearers had nothing to do but laze around in the sun all day.

But times are changing. Skin cancer, wrinkles, leathery skin— none of these are beautiful. Like their grandmothers, today's women are learning to stay inside and avoid the sun. You won't catch today's top models out in the sun without their sunscreen. Showing up on a job with a sunburn or over-tanned skin can cost a model a job. And if a model is tanned and bronze, she's probably wearing one of many bronzing gels now on the market. "None of the stars has a tan," says Laurence David, a California, dermatologist whose patients include such pale beau ties as Nicole Kidman and Kristen Dunst. "They know they won't get the parts they want if they have wrinkles."[1]

Dermatologists now believe that 80 percent of all damage done to skin occurs by age twenty, but a 1992 study indicates that only one in five teenagers wears sunscreen. If you receive as few as three blistering sunburns before the age of twenty, you're five times more likely to develop a melanoma, the deadliest of skin cancers, than someone who never got a sunburn. Pretty scary, right? Maybe it will scare you even more to realize that melanoma is the number one cancer among women ages twenty-five to twenty-nine.[2] So, for your own sake, cover up when you're in the sun!

Tap, tap, tap. (That's us rapping on your sun-tanned forehead). Time for a brief astronomy lesson:

There are two kinds of ultraviolet rays produced by the sun. The short rays, UVB, are the main cause of sunburn. These rays do the most damage between 10 a.m. and 2 p.m. The longer UVA rays shine down primarily in the morning and late afternoon.

Eighty percent of all ultraviolet rays can penetrate haze, light clouds, or even fog. They can "bounce up" from snow, sand, or water. You can be sunburned under a hat, an umbrella, or even in the shade. You can be burned through a wet tee shirt even if it's fifty degrees outside.

Got that? Don't mess around with ol' Mister Sun. If you are sunburned, apply cold compresses to your skin and take two aspirin every five hours. Calamine lotion or a hydrocortisone cream from the drug store will help cool your skin. If the skin bubbles and blisters, you have a second degree burn, and you need to see a doctor right away.

Even if you're not burned, Mister Sun's nasty ultraviolet rays dry out your top layer of skin, thicken the under layers, break down your skin's fibers, and even alter the DNA in your skin cells. Those UV rays can fry your hair and make it brittle, so wear a hat or scarf in the sun, especially if your hair is long, permed, bleached, or processed in anyway.

So what's a girl to do about that nasty sun? Wear protective stuff like hats and *sunscreen*. Laura tans easily (not a plus for a model!), so she wears a hat, a long-sleeved white shirt, and white cotton pants over her bathing suit to the beach. She even wears a full wet suit while windsurfing, boogie boarding, or water skiing, just to keep the sun off her body!

Don't forget, though, that sunscreens won't stop you from being burned. They simply slow the burning process and allow you more time in the sun than you would have had if you faced Mister Sun with your bare skin alone. For instance, if you're usually pink after twenty minutes in the sun, a lotion with an SPF (Sun Protection Factor) of 15 will let you stay out 15 times longer, or 300 minutes. But after 300 minutes, you'll turn pink.

Dermatologists recommend that everyone—even people with dark skin—wear a sunscreen with an SPF 15 every day, and put it on thick. Allow thirty minutes or so for the sunscreen to penetrate your skin, and reapply every two hours and after swimming. Some sunscreens, such as Bain de Soleil Sport Lotion and Coppertone Sport Dry Lotion, are waterproof. Sunscreens come in cream, lotion, gel, spray, and oil formulas.

Sunblocks screen out all the sun's rays. These are a must for girls with fair skin or those who are allergic to the sun. For the ultimate in protection, zinc oxide ointments are physical barriers often used by lifeguards and ski instructors. Now they (zinc oxide ointments, not lifeguards and ski instructors) even come in wild colors. Laura uses pink zinc on her lips — it looks like lipstick!

Moisturizing oils like baby oil and cocoa butters offer no protection from the sun. They do soften the skin, but if you're wearing them out in the sun you can get a nasty burn in less time than you think.

If you're feeling stubborn and you really want a tan, consider one of the sunless tanning products available, such as Clinique's Self-Tanning Formula, Estee Lauder's Self-Action Tanning Spray, or Clarins Self-Tanning Face Cream. These products contain dihydroxyacetone which combines chemically with the skin's amino acids to produce a darker skin tone. These products are not like the old "bronzers" that had to be reapplied everyday; instead they work year-round and develop a rapid "tan" on all skin types without sun. They don't wash off, and they fade naturally. Before using a self-tanner, be sure and read the directions on how to apply the product.

Major important note: Self-tanning products *do not* protect you from the sun. If you're using a self-tanning product and you go out in the sun, you still need to wear sun block or a sunscreen.

Mucho major important note to avoid embarrassment: After you've applied a self-tanning cream, be sure to wash your hands or you'll have orange palms. To give the backs of your hands a golden glow while keeping your palms clean, squirt a little extra formula on your legs and rub the backs of your hands there to pick up the excess.

If you're not into the tanned look, consider your pale beauty an asset. An entire crop of pale lovelies has sprung up, and you can set the standard among your friends.

Let's Get Personal

While we're talking about such personal things as showers, shaving, and sunbathing, we might as well discuss puberty, periods, perspiration, and protection.

As you know, you began to grow a woman's body when you were about nine years old. Your breasts began to develop, pubic hair began to grow, you shot up a few inches. You began to grow hair under your arms, and then the most obvious sign of womanhood occurred: You began to menstruate, to have your monthly period.

The entire process of puberty took about three years, and it was probably pretty gradual. What set it in motion? The hypothalamus gland, a tiny gland located at the base of your brain. It's the master control switchboard for the female hormone cycle, and while you're between the ages of eight and eighteen, the hypothalamus is responsible for making sure you become a mature woman. Congratulations, you're on your way!

Now this isn't the king of thing we usually talk about over the family dinner table, but when you reach puberty, you develop a new and obnoxiously different kind of sweat gland. Your body has two types: the smaller eccrine glands, of which you have a million or so, produce odorless sweat. But the larger apocrine glands, found in your armpits, ears, and private parts, produce an odor. The apocrine glands don't function until you reach puberty, then they spring into action and make up for lost time.

That's another reason it's important to take a bath or shower every day. Use a deodorant soap in the shower, and use a deodorant or antiperspirant for your underarms every day. Deodorants neutralize the odor of perspiration. Antiperspirants actually close off your skin's pores, so you *can't* sweat. Antiperspirants should be used only on your armpits because their main ingredient, an aluminum salt, may irritate the skin if used elsewhere on the body. Both antiperspirants and deodorants come in stick, spray, powder, cream, or liquid form.

By the way—it won't do any good to take a daily bath or shower unless your *clothes* are cleaned and/or well-aired after wearing. Odor can linger in your clothes, too!

Some girls worry that having their periods, or menstruating, causes an offensive body odor. If you take care of your body while you're menstruating and keep yourself as clean as possible, you shouldn't have to worry about odor. Odor is usually caused by growing bacteria, so keep yourself clean and change your tampons or sanitary napkins frequently.

Some girls look forward to beginning menstruation because it's an obvious sign they are growing up. One girl Angie knows proudly announced to her friends that her "friend" had come to stay, so she had to go out for "party favors"!

Other girls are frightened or worried that they'll be embarrassed or unprepared when menstrual bleeding begins. If you're worried, why not carry one of those slim "light days" panty-liners in your purse? You could keep it in a zippered pocket, or even in a plain white envelope. If you do begin your period away from home, the panty-liner will help you feel secure and give you time to get a sanitary napkin or tampon.

You may have seen television commercials about douches and feminine deodorants, but these products are not necessary for good hygiene. God designed your body to be "self-cleaning," and you do not have to douche after your monthly period to finish "cleaning yourself out." Your body cleans itself. Likewise, if you shower or bathe daily, you should not have to use feminine deodorants.

Facts and Fiction

- *You can't go swimming if you're on your period.*
- *It's awful. It's the curse.*
- *Boys can tell, you know. They can tell just by looking at you.*

All of the above are definitely not true. You shouldn't worry about menstruation, because "getting your period" is natural and normal. Probably every grown woman you know either has menstruated or still does it's a normal part of a woman's life.

When you were born, the ovaries inside your body contained all the eggs your body would ever need. The children you will bear will come from the three hundred thousand or so eggs inside your body right now. That's a wild thought, isn't it? God designed the entire process, and He knew what He was doing.

When the menstrual cycle begins, one egg is released from your ovaries each month, and it travels down the fallopian tube to the uterus, the organ where a baby may someday grow. As the egg travels, the lining of the uterus thickens, just as a mother bird feathers a nest to make it nice and soft for the eggs she will lay.

If the egg is united with a sperm from a man through sexual intercourse, it has everything it needs to become a baby. The embryo, or fertilized egg, nestles into the thick wall of the uterus. There it will grow for about nine months or until the baby is born.

If the egg is not fertilized, it disintegrates and the lush lining of the uterus is not needed. It sheds out of the uterus throughout the next five to seven days, resulting in "bleeding" through a woman's vagina.

Most women repeat this entire cycle every 27-30 days. The actual time of bleeding may be as short as one day or as long as eight days. Girls can begin to menstruate as early as nine years old or as late as sixteen.

Don't be worried if your periods are irregular in the first year. Many girls find that their menstrual cycle always varies a day or two, and other girls find theirs as punctual as clockwork. Dieting, obesity, extreme exercise, stress, or illness can throw your natural cycle off schedule.

Do not worry if your cycles are as short as twenty-one days or as long as forty-two days.

Do not worry if your period lasts only from one or two days, or as long as six to eight.

Do not worry if your periods are very light, or if you soak six to eight pads a day.

See a doctor if you are bleeding every day, or only once or twice a year after the first year.

See a doctor if you are bleeding more than six to eight days with every period.

See a doctor if your bleeding is heavy (more than six to eight pads), especially if you are weak or tired during your menstrual cycle.

Menstrual Protection

As you know, tampons are compressed materials worn *inside* the body. Are they safe? Yes. Millions of women use them every day. They allow better hygiene than pads; since the expelled material is held inside the body, bacteria and odor cannot form outside the body. Tampons also allow for greater freedom. You can swim, ride horses, do gymnastics, or practically *anything* while you are wearing a tampon.

The disadvantages of wearing a tampon arise if you do not change the tampon frequently. Years ago it was discovered that super-absorbent tampons, which could be worn for longer periods of time, encouraged the growth of bacteria inside the body and occasionally resulted in toxic shock syndrome. Some women died after contracting this disease, and those super-absorbent tampons were taken off the market.

If you wear a tampon, remember to change it every four to six hours. Never force a tampon into your body. If it is uncomfortable or painful, remove it. And always remove the last tampon you use each period. Some women find it easier to wear tampons for the first three days of a menstrual cycle when bleeding is heaviest, then they switch to a "light days" pad or panty liner for the remaining days.

Personal Protection

There is one final "p" to discuss in this section on personal subjects: personal protection.

Remember these things:

Your body is your own. No one has the right to touch or handle it without your permission.

Your feelings count. If you are uncomfortable in any situation, do something. Say something!

You have the right to say no if someone is pressuring you to perform a sexual act of any kind.

You should *run* from anyone who wants to touch you in a private area or who wants you to touch him or her in a private area.

There are people who want to help you. Find someone you can trust, and don't be afraid to say what's on your mind.

3
THE EYES HAVE IT

Claudia McClintock, another model, has eyes that sparkle with life and vitality. She has found that exercise is the key to overall health and beauty:

> Because I am a model, I felt compelled to join gyms, work out, and keep trim. But my efforts had the reverse effect, and I never knew why. I'd go twice to the gym and quit, reasoning that I was lazy. Then I came to the conclusion that as an Aussie born farm girl, nothing could substitute for natural, outdoor exercise. That's what I was used to. Physically, I'd burn the calories, while spiritually I was renewed and joyful within. That's what puts the sparkle in my eyes.

Wilhelmina, the former president of Wilhelmina Models, believes eyes are a woman's most important beauty asset: "Without lifting a finger or moving a muscle, a clever woman says more with her eyes than with her lips. Regardless of their size or shape, the eyes set the entire tone of who and what a woman is."[1]

The commonly accepted standard of beauty decrees that eyes be large and shining, with thick, long lashes, and delicately chiseled brows above. Whether or not your eyes measure up to this standard, you can help your eyes radiate with your own inner beauty.

Let's begin at the top and work down.

Just Browsing...

Your eyebrows, the thin lines of hair growing above your eyes, serve a double purpose. They keep dirt and perspiration from dripping down into your eyes, and they provide a pleasing frame for your eyes.

The most pleasing eyebrow shape is a delicate, neat curve. To rid your brows of excess hair, fetch your tweezers. You won't want to use a depilatory on your eyebrows — never allow any chemical near your eyes. Most women find that plucking stray eyebrow hair is simple and relatively painless.

Eyebrow plucking is easiest when your skin is fresh and softened from a warm shower or bath. Make sure the skin around your eyebrows is clean, then dip your tweezers in alcohol to sterilize them. Pluck the hairs that veer outside the clean sweep of your brows in quick, upward movements. When you are finished, apply antiseptic ointment or a drop of calamine lotion to the tweezed area to guard against infection.

Don't feel that your brows must look just like someone else's. Every face is different. Some girls have brows that are wonderfully bushy and quite striking. Other girls have more delicate, sparse brows. You can decide how you want your brows to look, but the primary purpose of plucking is to tweeze out stray hairs that veer away from the main sweep of your natural browline.

You can determine where your brows should begin and end with the pencil test. While looking in a mirror, hold a pencil vertically and rest the pencil against the right side of the bottom of your nose. The pencil will pass over the beginning of your eye and should also cross the beginning of your brow. Any hairs that remain on the left side of the pencil (over your nose) should be plucked from your right eyebrow.

Now, while keeping the pencil at the base of your nose, tilt it so that it directly crosses over the outer point of your eye. Notice where the pencil intersects your eyebrow. Any hairs that remain *past* the pencil should be plucked. Don't pluck your brow too short, because the shorter the brow, the smaller your eye will appear.

Don't allow the front part of your brow to drop below the back part and vice versa. After plucking, hold your pencil perfectly horizontal under your brow — the beginning and end of your brow should both touch the edge of the pencil. After you've perfectly plucked your right brow, repeat the procedure with your left.

When should you pluck your eyebrows? Laura suggests plucking before bed so any resulting redness will have time to disappear before you face the world.

If you feel your brows need color, don't use heavy eyebrow pencils. Often they are oil-based and merely mat the hairs together. Instead, if your brows are truly sparse or light, brush them with the brush from a nearly dried-up tube of mascara or with a colored powder. This will not only color them lightly, but will also thicken fine hairs.

One final hint: You can control unruly eyebrows by lightly spraying a soft toothbrush with hair spray or gel and immediately combing your brows upward and outward. A neat trick.

Eye Shadows

Blue eye shadow should be illegal. That's what Paula Begoun, a makeup artist, fervently believes. If you're complimented on your eye shadow, says Paula, you're not applying your makeup right.

Blue eye shadow was the rage years ago, but unless you want to look like you're wearing your mother's old makeup, look at the colors professional makeup artists apply to current fashion models. Most cosmetic ads list the makeup colors, and you can buy variations of those tones to fit your skin type and individual coloring.

When you apply eye shadow, use a small brush. If you want to use one color alone on your eyelid, choose a soft neutral color like tan or taupe, and apply it from your lashes to under your eyebrow. Bright colors should not be used as a single color. If you prefer a two-color design, use one color on the lid, and another color from the crease of the eyelid and slightly higher. Remember that light colors bring areas out, dark colors push areas back. You will probably want the darker color across the eyelid and the lighter color in the crease and to the brow.

If you choose a three-color scheme, apply one color on the inner two-thirds of the lid, another on the area from the crease to the brow, and the third color as a "wedge" from the crease to the outside of the eye on the back third of your lid. For instance, you can wear a pale tan on the lid (light colors bring out), a shimmery off-white under the brow, and a deep color in the wedge to make your eyes seem more deep-set.

Avoid placing too much eye shadow near the inner corner of your eyes. Always work from the inside out and add color as you move up and out from your pupils.

As you begin to choose makeup colors for your eyes, consider dressing your eyes the same way you'd dress your body. If your blush and lipstick are warm rusts and browns, your eye shadows should be from the same color family — peachy colors.

Not only should your eyes not clash with your face, don't let them clash with your clothes. That doesn't mean you have to wear a blue skirt with blue shadow and blue lipstick, but all colors have either warm (yellow) or cool (blue) undertones. Ideally, your makeup and clothes should be from the same color family and match your skin tone.

As you choose eye shadow colors, avoid colors that are more intense than you are. Make sure your eye makeup fits your circumstance. While Angie was doing research for a book about dating, she asked guys what they liked and didn't like in girls, and the guys had one common complaint: They hated it when girls wore too much makeup. Actually, guys don't want us not to wear makeup — and most of us look better with a little sprucing up. But guys want us to look like we're not wearing any (or much), and the fresh, natural look is what they find most appealing.

So if you're going to school, opt for gentle makeup choices and leave the dark eye shadows and heavy eyeliners in the drawer. Heavier makeup should be for special occasions and nighttime. Gaudy colors just don't look natural in daylight, and they look out of place at school and at the beach.

Eyeliners

Eyeliners, used to further define the eyes, are available in many forms: cream, stick, powder, and easy-to-apply pencils. Eyeliner should be applied after eye shadows and before mascara. Eyeliner is probably the most difficult eye makeup to apply because it requires a steady hand and a light touch. Too much eyeliner makes the eyes look hard.

When you line your eyelids, make sure the line is solid and even. To get your line close to your lashes, lift your eyelid slightly with your finger or raise your eyebrow. Practice painting thin lines beginning at the inner third of your eyelid, and thicken the line slightly as you near the outer third of your eyelid. When lining your lower lashes, line only the outer two-thirds of your eye with a softer color than that used on your eyelid. Make sure the two lines of your upper and lower lid meet at the outer corner of your eye. To soften a hard line, use an eye brush to smooth the color or brush a lighter eye shadow over the line to make it look more natural. Resist the temptation to paint on "wings." You're not Cleopatra.

Choose soft colors for eyeliner like brown, gray, or soft black. Laura recommends the L'Oreal "Le Crayon" eye pencil. It is soft, easy to apply, and stays on all day.

Mascara

Most girls tend to believe when applying mascara that more is better. But more mascara doesn't look like longer lashes, it only looks like more mascara. Besides, too much mascara can literally weigh your fragile lashes down and break them off.

There are basically three types of mascara: waterproof, water-soluble, and lash-lengthening. Waterproof mascara may be fine for swimmers or girls who cry *a lot,* but to remove it you must wipe and pull at your lashes. In our opinion, the disadvantages of waterproof mascara aren't worth the advantage. Nobody cries that much.

Water-soluble mascara works well and is easy to remove. Best of all, if a chunk of it falls into your eye, it will dissolve, not stick around and scratch your eye (another hazard of waterproof mascara!).

Lash-lengthening mascaras usually contain fibers that supposedly lengthen lashes. But these fibers can drift into your eye and cause damage.

So which type of mascara do we recommend? Water-soluble. It's safe, beautiful, and easy to remove. Best of all, if you make a mistake when applying it, it's gone with one swipe of a moistened cotton swab.

Laura always uses Maybelline Great Lash, and she says it's a favorite of several makeup artists in New York City. It is not expensive and works great!

To make a tube of mascara last longer, buy a mascara with a smaller brush. The size of the brush really doesn't matter when you're applying mascara, but a larger brush allows more air into the tube, and additional air dries mascara out faster. Mascaras also dry out more quickly if you "pump" the brush into the tube when you're applying mascara. You're not necessarily getting more mascara on the brush, but you are pumping air into the tube. You should always throw away your tube of mascara after six months because dark, moist mascara tubes can collect bacteria that could get into your eye. And never share your mascara!

What color should you wear? Take a cue from your hair. Fair blondes and redheads should probably wear brown mascara. Dark-haired brunettes can wear black. No one should wear electric blue mascara. It's distracting. People will notice your eyelashes—not you.

Angie admits she was a little shocked when a makeup artist from Estee Lauder suggested that she wear navy blue mascara, but after trying it she discovered the navy mascara was dark enough to add definition to her eyes, but not as overpowering as black mascara. It's a nice effect and the mascara looks natural, not blue.

On the other hand, the sales girl wanted to sell a tube of navy mascara . . . so Angie mostly wears brown or brown/black for every day.

By the way, if you have sensitive eyes, you might react to certain brands of mascara. Angie remembers one time when she was driving in traffic and the glare of the sun made her eyes water. When her mascara began to melt, it stung her eyes so badly that she had to weave through traffic and pull off to the side of the road where she could safely wipe her eyes. She looked like a black-eyed monster after that, but she learned to avoid that brand of mascara. If a certain brand of mascara stings your eyes, try something else.

Under the Eyes

Beautiful eyes don't stop with the bold makeups like eyeliners and eye shadows. The fragile skin under the eyes often needs help, too.

If you are prone to dark circles under the eyes, you may use a concealer stick or cream to cover them, but such concealers shouldn't be applied in a half-circle under the entire eye area. You'll end up with raccoon eyes. Instead, make three little dots just under the inside corner of the eye, and blend the concealer down and out. Always be gentle when rubbing skin in this area. Some beauty experts even suggest that you apply makeup here with a soft makeup sponge or your ring finger because it is the weakest finger and less likely to stretch your skin.

What causes "circles" under the eyes? The skin under your eyes is thin and delicate, and the tiny blood vessels in the skin are visible, giving a dark blue tone to the skin. When you are tired or sick, the circles look even darker because less blood is going to your face, and the blood vessels under the eye area stand out even more than usual. Dark circles under the eyes can also be caused by sun damage, so this area should always be protected by a sunscreen or sunglasses when you are outdoors.

Glass Can Be Class

"I'll never have pretty eyes as long as I have to wear glasses!"

Not true. Lasses who wear glasses can make the best of wearing fabulous frames.

Ask a friend to help you with this. Have her look at your eyes without glasses, then put on your glasses. Do your lenses magnify your eyes or make them look smaller?

If your glasses magnify your eyes, choose soft colors for your eye shadows and eyeliner, and avoid a heavy coat of mascara. If your glasses make your eyes look smaller, increase your makeup colors and definition, but be careful to avoid hard edges. In either case, make sure your blush begins below the edge of your glasses.

When you're considering what sort of frames to get for your glasses, hold a pair of frames in front of you and draw an imaginary horizontal line through the center of the frames, where you'd expect to see the center of your eyes. If the bridge (the place where they join together) of the frames is high above the imaginary line, they are high-bridge frames. If it is not far from your imaginary line, they are low-bridge.

If you want to make your short nose seem longer, buy high-bridge frames. If you wish to make a long nose shorter, buy a pair of low-bridge frames. A dark bridge will make a wide nose seem narrower. Decorations on the outer edges of the frames will draw a viewer's eye out, away from a prominent nose.

Have fun with your frames. Don't settle for the usual colors. If you're a pale blonde, consider rose, blue, green, or tortoise-shell frames. If you have olive skin or are a brunette, try brown, plum, rose, or blue frames. Redheads look great in tortoiseshell, green, coral, brown, and amber frames; and girls with black skin and/or hair could try rose, purple, or amber frames.

There are several designer frames on the market that are a lot of fun. So if you have to wear glasses, see them as an opportunity to make your own fashion statement!

Healthy, Happy Eyes

Your eyes are fragile instruments, but if you take care of them, they ought to bring you the world in living color throughout your lifetime. If you're doing close work like needlepoint, watching television, reading, or working at a computer terminal, stop every twenty minutes or so and focus on an object in the distance. This will relax your focusing muscles. Remember to blink your eyes occasionally to allow the eye's natural lubrication to do its job, and your eyes will thank you if you close your eyes for a few seconds to let your eyelids lubricate and shelter your tired eyes.

If your eyes become bloodshot, they've probably been irritated by allergies, eyestrain, pollution, a lack of sleep, or smoke. The tiny blood vessels in your eyes have expanded and filled up with blood in an attempt to bring more oxygen to your eyes. If this happens to you, wash your eyes with an isotonic solution like Blinx. Other eye drops like Clear and Brite and Murine Plus Eye drops contain tetrahydrozoline, an agent that shrinks swollen blood vessels.

Just as sun can fry your skin, it can also damage your eyes. Sunburns of the eye are serious and often do not show up for twelve to twenty-four hours. If you've been in the sun and wake at night with burning pain in your eyes, see an eye doctor immediately.

To prevent sun damage to your eyes, wear sunglasses chosen with safety, not fashion, as your primary consideration. Stay away from high-fashion colored lenses in pink, orange, yellow, and blue —they let in too much sunlight. When you're shopping for sunglasses, try on a pair and look in the mirror. If you can see your eyes through the lenses, the glasses are not dark enough to protect your eyes.

4
MAKEUP MAGIC

Ali Winslow, another model and a friend of Laura's, once hated the structure of her face:

> I had huge teeth and huge eyes when I was growing up. I got teased a lot. When I grew up, I realized they were my strongest features and I play them up with makeup now that I'm a model. I chose to have short hair because now my small face and huge eyes don't get lost behind a lot of hair.

The word *cosmetics* comes from an ancient Greek word *kosmos*, meaning "adornment." Cosmetics are supposed to help people notice your beauty — not the makeup. You don't want people to notice your furiously blushing cheeks or your electric green eyelids—you want them to notice the overall effect of your makeup, a pleasing picture of you. "The purpose of makeup," says Heloise of *Hints from Heloise* fame, "is to minimize or conceal flaws—not to make you look painted."[1]

Cosmetics, correctly applied, can give you a sense of confidence. Every girl feels better when she knows she looks her best.

The Basis of Makeup: Foundation
Many young girls don't wear foundation, or wear it only on

special occasions when they are striving for a "fully made up" look. But foundation can do a lot for you. First, it gives your powder makeups like eye shadows and blush something to cling to on your face. Second, it evens out any blotchy areas on your skin and covers up red areas where skin problems are beginning to erupt. A well-applied coat of foundation can make your skin look dewy and smooth, as well as guard your fragile face from the sun's dangerous ultraviolet rays.

You may think foundation is a no-no because it will clog your pores, but foundation can actually *protect* your pores from pollution and grime. Most foundations are now designed not to clog pores (they're labeled "non-comedogenic"), and many come with a sunscreen. Even those which don't contain sunscreen have a natural sunscreen protection factor of four.

When shopping for the perfect foundation, don't try the color on your hand or wrist or even your cheek. Test the color on your bare facial skin at a spot midway between the corner of your lower lip and your jawline. The right shade will seem to disappear into your skin, not stand out with rough edges.

If you're in a drug store where there are no samples or testers, hold a couple of bottles next to your face and choose a color a few shades lighter than you think you would wear (colors are more concentrated and darker in the bottle). If the match is not perfect, the next time you buy a bottle, buy a darker shade and mix the two.

Don't buy foundation thinking that it will enable you to lighten or darken your skin. You want an even, neutral base for your makeup, not a Halloween mask.

There are several different types of foundation available. *Oil-free* foundations come in two different forms. One is a watery mixture of talc, water, alcohol, and coloring agents. The second formulation is a creamy blend of water, propylene glycol, and waxes.

Creamy oil-free makeup glides on well, but is very heavy. Both types of oil-free makeup dry quickly, which means mistakes are harder to correct. The watery formulation with alcohol may dry your skin.

Water-based foundations are light and easy to apply, but they contain oil and may develop a shine after hours of wear. *Oil-based* foundations are thicker, heavier, and greasier. They tend to look heavy on the face.

How can you tell if your foundation is oil or water-based? Look at the list of ingredients. If oil is the first ingredient listed, it's an oil-based foundation.

The final type of foundation is *pancake makeup,* an oil-free foundation used mainly for theatrical purposes. If you try out for the school play, you're likely to get your face slathered with pancake makeup. It's heavy and definitely not for everyday wear.

What foundation do we recommend? A creamy water-based foundation. Teenagers typically don't need extra oil on their skin, and while your mother may love her oil-based foundation, you're likely to be happier without the extra oil.

To apply foundation, first, cleanse your skin. If you use a concealer at the inside corners of your eyes, use your gentle ring finger to blend the concealer in this area of fragile skin. Always pat your skin; never pull or wipe when applying any kind of makeup.

Now dot the foundation on the skin in the middle of your forehead, on your nose and chin, and under your eyebrows. A few little dots will do the job. Use your fingers, a dry nylon sponge, or a damp natural sponge to blend the foundation outward over your skin. Don't forget to put a light coat of foundation on your eyelid. This will give your eye shadow something to adhere to.

Don't feel you have to thickly coat your entire face with foundation. There should be no "line of demarcation" on your jawbone — in other words, no one should be able to tell where your foundation application begins and ends. Never, ever, apply foundation on your neck.

If you have a blemish that foundation won't cover, use a small eyeliner brush to apply a concealer that matches your skin. The small brush will enable you to work directly on the small area. Blend any excess concealer away from the blemish using the brush. Do not cover the blemish with a lot of powder or it will look dry.

Wear foundation well, and it will become an easy step in your makeup routine. Skip the foundation, though, if you're planning to go to the gym for an afternoon of sweating, and remember to take foundation off before going to bed. Your face deserves a rest, too.

Powder

Unless your skin is really oily, you probably won't need to purchase or wear face powder. If you have to wear makeup all day, though, you might enjoy a "powdering" in the afternoon, when your face's natural oils begin to shine through your foundation.

Don't be overzealous; some natural glow is appealing.

We recommend loose face powder, applied with a brush or velour puff, more than the pressed powders which come in a compact because pressed powders contain wax. Why wax your face when you can apply a light dusting of fresh powder easily ? (Pressed powders do offer an advantage if you're away from home and need to powder your nose and forehead. A pressed powder compact travels easily.)

Blushing

Throw away those too-small brushes that come with the pressed blush you buy. Your makeup brush should fit the area of skin being brushed, and your cheeks need a bigger brush than those scrawny things that come in makeup kits. You can buy an inexpensive set of makeup brushes in all sizes at the drug store.

The most obvious mistake girls make in makeup application is brushing two large red blotches on their cheeks. Blush should look natural, not like two crimson racing stripes.

When you apply blush, look into the mirror and draw an imaginary line straight down from your pupil. Now imagine a horizontal line extending from the tip of your nose. Your "blush" should go no further down your face than the imaginary intersection of those two lines. Now place your blush brush high on your cheekbone and brush downward toward that imaginary intersection, applying color gently. Don't brush up and away — that encourages the stripe effect. The blushed area should be no more than one and a half inches wide and you should never be able to tell where you started or stopped your blush brush.

Never apply blush around your eye, below your mouth, or near the "laugh lines" that form at the outside corners of your eyes. Never blush your nose, your forehead, your hairline, or your chin. Cheeks blush. Chins don't.

Lipstick and Lip Liner

Before applying lipstick or lip liner, Laura suggests that you first apply a natural lip gloss, let it sit for a while, and then blot it with a tissue. This will moisten your lips and prepare them for things to come.

When lining your lips, always follow the actual outline of your lips. If you are tempted to make your mouth appear bigger by lining outside your lip line, when your lipstick wears off (and it will), you'll look like you missed your mouth!

The fad of wearing dark lip liner and lighter lipstick has passed, thank goodness. Though your liner may be a shade darker, dark brown lip liner and pink lipstick just doesn't look good. It never did. Paula Begoun says, "Lip liner stopped being an obvious dark, brown, definite line around the mouth in 1978. Lip liner for contemporary fashion should not show obviously at all."[2] Choose lip pencils in natural lip colors.

If your lipstick seems to "bleed" after a while, avoid greasy lipsticks and lip liners or consider lining your mouth smaller than it actually is. To seal your lipstick, Laura offers this model's trick: After applying lipstick, place a thin layer of tissue lightly over your lips and use a fluffy makeup brush to lightly brush them with loose face powder. Gently lift the tissue. You're beautiful.

Makeup Tips and Tidbits

☐ If a cosmetics package has been opened, do not buy it.

☐ Apply your cosmetics to a squeaky clean face with clean hands.

☐ Never put cosmetics on broken or irritated skin.

☐ Don't share cosmetics with your friends.

☐ Don't use store testers on your lips or eyes.

☐ Don't store makeup in heat or direct sunlight.

☐ If a makeup makes your skin break out or sting, discontinue use and try another brand.

☐ Buy a new tube of mascara every six months.

☐ Expensive makeups sold in department stores may not be any better than those sold at your local grocery store. If a product works for you, don't spend extra money for a fancier version.

☐ "Hypo-allergenic" usually means that a product has no fragrance, lanolin, or other ingredient that commonly causes allergic reactions. But if your skin is very sensitive, any ingredient at all could cause a reaction, so don't assume that a hypo-allergenic makeup *can't* cause an allergic reaction.

☐ Cosmetics that are labeled "non-comedogenic" do not contain ingredients that will clog pores and encourage comedones—that is, blackheads. Look for non-comedogenic foundations, powders, blushes, and sunscreens.

☐ Dermablend, another makeup designed to hide scars, bruises, and other disfiguring marks, is sold in fine department stores. You don't have to blindly accept a disfiguration. Cosmetics may not only help you, they may change your life by increasing your confidence.

Makeup Balance

Part of the art of wearing makeup successfully is choosing cosmetics that are properly balanced: the right look at the right place at the right time. Paula Begoun says:

> Balance refers back to the clothing confusion between wearing a business suit or jogging suit to the wrong occasion. Makeup coincides with those outfits the same way because it is part of the outfit. Fully applied makeup with a jogging outfit is as inappropriate as no makeup with a business suit or an evening dress. . . . If you wouldn't wear a pair of high heels with your jogging outfit, don't wear an evening-type makeup with it either.[3]

The art of makeup is the flow of color and line on the face from one point to another so the viewer's eye never rests on any particular aspect of the application. Overdoing the eyes with black liner and dark eye shadows and not balancing it out with strong lipstick and blush will not look finished. The same is true for lots of blush color and no eye shadow or lipstick.

Never in history has it been easier or healthier for women to wear makeup. In Elizabethan times, women rubbed their skin with *ceruse*, a white paste that contained lead. Not only did this lead enter their bloodstreams, but the paste caused the skin to corrode and crack. Other women swallowed gravel, ashes, coal dust, or tallow candles in an effort to obtain white skin. Some eighteenth-century women used oil of vitriol, an acid stronger than battery acid, to strip away their skin's outer layer.[4]

Today's makeups are not only more natural-looking, many are actually good for you. So wear your makeup well.

5

YOUR BEST BEAUTY ASSET: YOUR SMILE

Model Sara Richmond remembers a time when she didn't feel like smiling:

> In high school, I hated having red hair and being called "carrot top" so I tried to make my hair blonde. Now I thank God that He gave me red hair, and that He's made each of us different. What I thought was my worst attribute has become my greatest blessing.

We discussed lipsticks and lip liners in Chapter 4, but a smile is worth a thousand words, and at least a chapter of its own.

Never underestimate the power of a smile. Of course, as Shakespeare said, "One may smile, and smile, and be a villain," but usually a smile says, 'I'm friendly. I'd like to get to know you." That kind of openness will make you beautiful!

It's not appropriate to walk around wearing a broad smile all the time—people would think you are crazy. But a warm and friendly smile can turn a sullen woman into a beautiful one, and it can be *the most important thing you wear.*

A smile can also make you feel better. According to psychologist R. B. Zajonc of the University of Michigan at Ann Arbor, there could be a physiological explanation for the link between a happy expression and a positive mental attitude. Says author David Lewis, "There is good reason for supposing that a happy face can boost your mood, not only by triggering the release of 'happy' chemicals in the brain but also by encouraging a relaxed and agreeable response from others. . . .[A smile's] usual effect is to increase the chances that others will like us."[1]

Those Pearly Whites: Part of a Healthy Smile

If you want to have a great-looking smile, take care of your teeth. Your toothbrush should be among your most important beauty brushes.

After you eat, tiny food particles remain in your mouth and lodge in the pits and crevasses of your teeth. While they remain there, they react with the saliva in your mouth and attack the enamel of your teeth. This attack can easily result in tooth decay and gum infection, so brush your teeth regularly and learn how to use dental floss. Flossing goes where no toothbrush has gone before, and it will help you maintain a healthy smile.

You don't have to get cavities, you know. It's very possible that your teeth can last a lifetime without problems if you take good care of them.

Proper nutrition is also important for healthy teeth. Foods rich in calcium, vitamin D, magnesium, vitamin A, niacin, Vitamin B-complex, zinc, and vitamin C will help. Instead of chewing gum and candy bars, reach for sesame seeds, cheese, brazil nuts, sunflower seeds, walnuts, and peanuts. Don't forget to drink lots of milk!

Regular dental care is a must. Your dentist will show you how to brush and floss your teeth, and he'll indicate spots in your mouth you may have missed in your regular cleaning. He will also check to make sure you have no cavities or other serious dental problems.

Some experts say the type of foods we eat has a huge effect on dental health. For instance, sticky foods that cling to our teeth cause greater damage than sweet treats that are swallowed and seen no more. So if you're eating raisins, chewy candy, dates, or bananas, brush your teeth right away. Whenever possible, avoid soft drinks made with sugar.

Orthodontics: Tools for a Healthy Smile

If you were born with a beautiful smile, rejoice. But if you were like Angie, born with too many large teeth and a too-small jaw, you may have to correct your smile with orthodontics: braces. Braces aren't anything like they were years ago, and they're cropping up on mouths of kids, teenagers, and adults alike. Correctly spaced teeth are important not only for your smile and your self-confidence, but for the proper development of your body. If your teeth are badly out of line, you may have problems chewing, cleaning your teeth, even speaking well. You may find yourself insecure and reluctant to smile in public.

A national survey of kids ages six to eleven found that only 46 percent had teeth that properly fit together. All of the others — fifty-four kids out of one hundred—could have benefited from braces. Twenty-nine out of one hundred *definitely* needed braces to correct a severe problem.[2]

When Angie wore braces, there wasn't much to the process. The orthodontist made a plaster cast of her crooked teeth (in her case, an extreme overbite), then pulled six teeth so the few that remained would have room in her mouth. A shiny metal band was placed around each tooth and cemented into place, then a "guiding wire" was looped through each tooth band to string all the teeth together. A pair of tiny rubber bands was the force that pulled the teeth to their proper place.

Once a month Angie went to have her braces checked, and the rubber bands got smaller and smaller. Her mouth was always tender and sore for a couple of days after her visit to the orthodontist, but never was it unbearable. She experienced only one hour or so of genuine horror: One night while Angie was home alone, she got the top of her tongue caught in the wire at the front of her braces. She couldn't free herself, and when her mother came home from choir practice, Angie ran out into the hall, pointing wildly at her trapped tongue and tried to explain: "Thy thot thy thonge thought thin thy thaces."

Angie's mom called the orthodontist, who arranged to meet them at a local shopping center, halfway between his house and theirs. At ten o'clock at night, Angie knelt in her nightgown and robe in front of the car's headlights in a parking lot while cars whizzed by on the highway. The orthodontist expertly extracted her tongue with one flip of a dental instrument, and the adventure was over. After eighteen months, the braces came off, Angie got a retainer, and her new smile was worth every second of soreness. Laura not only wore braces, but endured mouth surgery and two retainers. "The whole ordeal," she says, "lasted over three years, but it was worth every bit of it!" Most girls who wear braces feel the same way.

There is a wide variety of orthodontic treatments available now. The old "tin grin" braces have been replaced by lighter, almost invisible materials. Some orthodontic devices are removable, some are worn part-time outside the mouth, and others are permanently attached to the teeth for two to three years. Braces today can be formed of plastic that blends into the color of the teeth instead of the bright chrome that Angie and Laura wore.

If braces are in your future, you should know about the following improvements in orthodontics:

☐ Metal braces today now come with hard to detect mini brackets for the "guiding wire" that can fit on either the front or back of teeth.

☐ Plastic braces aren't as noticeable because they're clear. But the disadvantage to plastic braces is that they are not as strong as metal and are easily stained by food.

Ceramic braces are translucent, with smoother edges that soothe and ease irritation to gums. Ceramic braces are more durable than plastic, and more expensive.

☐ The rubber bands that power tooth movement are now available in wild colors like red, black, and neon hues. Your orthodontist can now match your rubber bands to your prom dress.

☐ Dental care is even more important when you're wearing braces. You should brush after *every* meal (carry a portable toothbrush), and avoid sticky, crunchy, sweet, or hard foods. These are hard to remove from your teeth and can bend the fragile wires guiding your teeth.

☐ If your gums or the inside of your mouth becomes sore or irritated by your braces, rinse the inside of your mouth with a glass of warm saltwater. Don't swallow.

☐ When you're wearing braces, make the most of your eye makeup. Keep lipstick colors neutral by avoiding rich reds, glossy colors, and frosted shades.

☐ Retainers, the mouth-shaped plastic piece that reminds

your newly repositioned teeth to stay in place, are now available in cool colors or with embossed designs. When such a colorful retainer is on your lunch tray (they must be removed for meals), you'll be less likely to throw it into the trash can with your garbage.

Whatever program your orthodontist chooses for you, don't be tempted to "rush" your treatment. Dr. Stephen Goodman, a New York periodontal specialist, warns that "if the stresses are too great, you can end up with loose teeth."[3] So trust your orthodontist, and don't mess with your program or beg for early release. It takes time to make a permanent change (usually twelve to thirty months), but the results will be worth it.

Bad Breath Blues

Halitosis is bad breath's formal name, and everyone suffers from it once in a while. What causes it? Well, there's stale "morning breath" which strikes all of us every morning. Bad breath can also be caused by spicy foods or beverages, infection in the throat, tonsils, or sinuses, bad gums, an upset stomach, or smoking.

If you ever cough up small white lumps that smell to high heaven, these are most likely tonsil stones, or tonsiliths. Some people have small openings, or crypts, in their tonsils, and these openings can collect food. Over time, the food decays and the material becomes compacted until you cough if up or swallow it.

You can remove these stones manually (search the internet for methods), or you can take the somewhat drastic step of having your tonsils removed. Not everyone has cryptic tonsils, but many people do.

How do you get rid of ordinary bad breath? For starters, you might try one of the many mouthwashes on the market, brush your tongue, or chew a sprig of mint or parsley. (Yes, I am referring to the parsley that often comes as decoration on a plate in a restaurant. You can eat it, and it's good for you!)

If breath mints and mouthwashes don't seem to work for you, the problem may spring from your stomach. Nutrition-oriented doctors often suggest that people with halitosis take a tablespoon of apple cider vinegar just before each meal. This will help your digestion and should knock out bad breath.

There is also the possibility that bad breath is caused by food literally rotting in the mouth. If you don't brush your teeth soon after every meal, food particles remain in the mouth and begin to putrefy. So brush your teeth. If you have a choice between reaching for a mouthwash or a toothbrush after every meal, the toothbrush will do more to cure bad breath.

If you're in a restaurant or some place where you absolutely can't brush your teeth, take a sip from your water glass and discreetly swish the water in your mouth, then swallow. You may be able to at least partially flush your mouth clean.

The Words You Leave Behind

We can't leave this chapter without addressing one last aspect of your mouth: your words. Have you ever stopped to think how your speech influences your beauty? Whether it is right or wrong, people do judge you by your words.

We're not talking about whether you choose to use slang or twelve-syllable words. We want to focus on what you say and how you say it. Do you guard your tongue against ugly words and retorts? Do you allow your tongue to put others down? Is anger part of the true spirit of beauty?

If you want to be beautiful from the inside out, consider what you allow to come out of your mouth. Speech or conversation that contains bitter anger, gossip, backbiting words, or cursing is not attractive or beautiful. And what good is a lovely face if what comes out of it isn't so lovely? Don't let peer pressure make you say "cool" things that are really nasty or mean.

Why not let your words be helpful, truthful, and sincere? Offer help when your friends are hurting, comfort the girl at school who's in pain, and encourage your friends with hope when they're depressed. *That's* being beautiful.

Sometimes it's easy to rattle off any dumb thing that comes into our heads. It's tempting to be like everyone else and use the vulgar expressions that we hear a thousand times a day on television, at school, and at the movies. But to be truly beautiful from the inside out, we have to do what isn't easy. We have to rise above the crowd and be different.

There's one more beautiful thing that can come from your mouth, and it goes perfectly with a smile: *laughter.* A good laugh works your heart, lungs, and chest muscles. Laughter chases stress right out the door. Best of all, laughter makes us and those around us—feel better.

So go ahead and laugh. This business of being beautiful isn't that serious.

6
SWEET FEET AND FAB FINGERS

Model Deborah remembers great advice from her mother:

> My mom told me to push my cuticles back after I
> bathe or shower because that's when they are soft.
> I use a washcloth or fingernail to push them back,
> then I apply petroleum jelly. If you do this, you
> will never need to cut your cuticles.

"It's very important as a model to have clean, manicured hands at all times," Laura says. "I never know when my hands will be in a shot or when I'll be asked to do a tight cropped shot of my hands holding a particular product."

No matter what impression you want to create, the state of your hands and nails tells how much you really care about your appearance.

Nails: How They Grow

Your finger and toenails are made of *keratin*, the same tough substance as your hair. But while hair is a long narrow sheath of keratin, your nails are keratin plates designed to protect the tender tips of your active hands and feet.

Like hair, a nail is composed of many parts. The visible part of your nail is called the *nail plate*. It is white in color, but looks pink because it lies on the nail bed, which contains tiny blood vessels and nerves.

The nail plate extends and grows outward from the root of the nail, which lies under the *lunule,* the pale half-moon shape at the base of your nail. Under the nail root lies a group of cells called *the matrix.* The matrix is very important because injury to this area, whether from malnutrition or hitting your hand with a hammer, can slow down the growth of the nail. Trauma, such as a blow or catching your finger in a door, can lead to the temporary or even permanent loss of a nail.

Surrounding and overlapping the base of the nail is the *cuticle,* a group of dead skin cells whose purpose is to keep dirt and bacteria away from the fragile matrix and nail bed.

Can you help your matrix produce long, lovely nails? Yes. You may not realize it, but your nails grow continuously. Nail growth begins at the matrix and moves forward toward the free edge of the nail. The average adult's nails grow one-eighth of an inch per month. Toenails grow more slowly, but they grow thicker and harder. Toenails are tough, and they need to be. Your feet can take some pretty hard knocks.

Your nails grow faster right before your monthly menstrual period and during warm weather (a summer bonus!). If a nail is injured, it will grow faster in the recovery period. The nails on your dominant hand (your right hand, if you're right-handed) grow faster than your other hand, and if you're a pianist or typist your nails may grow faster than the average person's. Scientists think that people with active fingers grow nails faster because pressure on their fingertip pads increases circulation to the nail bed. So if you want to grow your nails quickly, try tapping or typing!

There are no brush-on or rub-in products available that will actually stimulate nail growth, for nail growth begins internally. However, good nutrition will help, just as it aids your hair. And since nails and hair are both made of keratin, the same foods that improve your hair will also promote strong, healthy nails!

If you want to eat for pretty hair and nails, remember to focus on protein, magnesium, vitamin B-6, folic acid, and biotin. You'll find these ingredients in cheese, eggs, fish, meat, milk, yogurt, nuts, sunflower seeds, oats, brown rice, and wheat germ.

Feet Facts

You will take more than seven thousand steps in an average day and walk over 115,000 miles in your lifetime — that's five times around the globe. If you weigh one hundred thirty-five pounds, you'll put four hundred pounds of pressure on each foot as you walk. In an average day, your feet will release one cup of water as sweat!

Feet are definitely underappreciated. Each of your feet has twenty-six bones, fifty-six ligaments, thirty-eight muscles, 72,000 nerve endings, and 250,000 sweat glands. Pretty impressive, huh?

Our feet take a pounding throughout our lives. We walk, run, and sit on them. We kick with them, push with them, and even use them for picking things up off the floor. It's too bad, but feet just don't get any respect.

Take time to pamper your feet. For the best feet in town, first make sure your shoes fit properly. Give the high heels a rest, too. When you're not wearing shoes, 65 percent of your weight is carried on your heels, 35 percent on the forefoot. When you wear high heels, the balance shifts and your poor forefeet are stuck with the load.

Says Laura, "I've seen ruined feet with calluses and bunions on young girls who wore high heels frequently." Save the spiked heels for special occasions, and stick to lower heels for everyday wear.

Your feet will thank you if you never insert them into anything but clean socks and hose. Don't romp around the neighborhood in bare feet, and don't borrow or lend shoes. Even at the pool or beach, wear plastic sandals or those great new "aqua shoes" that protect and cushion your feet.

Just as you should wash your body every day, wash your feet, too. Don't forget to soap them in the bath or shower (don't slip!), and in warm weather sprinkle cornstarch or foot powder in your shoes to absorb perspiration. If the skin on your feet is dry and cracked or peeling, treat your feet to a daily dose of moisturizing lotion. If your feet ache after a long day, soak them in warm water sprinkled with Epsom salts, then follow with a cool soak.

If you don't have time for a soak, Laura suggests that you simply elevate your feet when you get home from a busy day. If only for a few minutes, it really helps!

Pretty Pedicures

We'll start with the feet, because the perfect pedicure should be performed *before* the perfect manicure. You're less likely to mess up your fingernails if your toenails are done first.

Your toenails grow fastest in warm weather, so you'll need to give yourself a pedicure every two weeks in summertime, and every three to four weeks in the winter.

When giving yourself a pedicure, begin by removing old nail polish with a cotton ball. Then cut and shape your nails. Toenails should be shaped straight across and trimmed with toenail clippers if nails extend beyond the tip of the toe. Buff the edges of the nails smooth.

After buffing, soak your feet in soap and water for five minutes. This will not only soften your feet but your cuticles, too. After five minutes, remove your feet and use the flat end of an orangewood stick to gently push your cuticles back. Now, while your feet are still soft and moist, use a heavy emery board or pumice stone to rub off any dry skin or calluses on your toes or feet.

Dry your feet, and follow with an application of creamy lotion on the tops and bottoms of your feet. Be careful not to get any lotion on your toenails—keep them clean for the polish that will follow. (Once a week it's a good idea to apply a heavy cream to your feet and sleep in socks. It sounds messy, but it will keep your feet soft and supple!)

Now that your feet are smooth, buff your nails from side to side until they shine. Then put tissues in between your toes to separate and prevent smearing during polishing. Next, apply the base coat and polish. If you are right-handed, begin with the small toe of your left foot; do the opposite if you are left-handed. Remember, toes look best in bright colors!

Finish with a top coat, remove the tissues between your toes, and wait at least one hour before going to bed or putting on shoes or socks. You don't want to get nail polish everywhere. When your toenails are very dry, apply another coat of creamy lotion and rub it into your cuticles.

Foot Problems

Corns are little circular lumps that appear on the feet, particularly on the big toe. They are lumps of dead skin cells, usually the result of pressure or friction. (They can be caused by wearing heels that are too tall. Try to wear heels no higher than one inch.) They are not painful or serious, and you may never have a problem with them. But they aren't very pretty.

To reduce your corns, try dabbing some baby oil on the corn

and soaking your feet in warm water. When the skin has softened somewhat, rub the corn gently with a Buf Puf or a pumice stone. Even if you wear the corn away, it may come back, so make "corn buffing" a regular part of your beauty routine.

Calluses are a painless thickening of skin on the ball of your foot where there is friction. Wearing shoes that are too tight or too loose may encourage calluses. Use a pumice stone or a chemical slougher to wear calluses away. Do not cut a callus with a razor blade, and don't remove the entire callus — that thickened skin is there for protection. If a callus causes pain or is hot or red, see a podiatrist.

If you've ever gone skating with too-thin socks, you know about *blisters*. If you develop a blister on your heel or foot, clean the area with alcohol, and gently puncture the raised blister with a sterile needle. After the fluid has drained, apply an antibiotic ointment and cover the blister with a bandage. Don't remove the dead skin. It is still needed for protection.

Plantar warts appear on the sole of the foot. These look like thick calluses, but are usually sensitive to pressure and are painful during walking. Also called *verruca plantaris*, plantar warts can only be removed by a physician or podiatrist. If you suspect you have one, don't neglect it. They are caused by viruses, and they can spread.

Ingrown toenails cause pressure, pain, redness, and swelling around the nail bed. They are usually caused by improper toenail clipping or by wearing pointy-toed shoes. Picking at toenails, ripping, or biting them can contribute to ingrown toenails, so cut your toenails straight across and don't pick at them. If you find you have an ingrown toenail, first soak your foot in warm salty water for about twenty minutes, then try to cut the nail so it's straight across, not angled. Apply an antibiotic cream. If this treatment doesn't ease the inflammation, see a doctor or podiatrist.

Whatever you do for an ingrown toenail, don't listen to the old wives' tale about cutting a V in the center of your toe. Toenails won't "grow together"; they grow from bottom to top only.

Big feet aren't really a physical problem, but when Angie was growing up, she thought they were. When you're tall, you usually have big feet to match, and it takes quite a mental effort to say, "These are my feet. They match my body. I can learn to feel good about them." Ha. When Angie was sixteen, she couldn't say that.

Your feet will stop growing when you are about eighteen,

though you may need larger shoes someday if you gain weight. So whatever size your feet become, learn how to make them look their best and realize that they are the right size for you.

It's a Shoe-in!

You can have the prettiest feet in the world, but if they're stuck in a pair of ratty shoes, the entire effect of your appearance is ruined. If you spend hours planning the perfect outfit, don't forget to plan the right pair of shoes, too!

As a general rule (though there are always exceptions), the longer the skirt length, the shorter the shoe's heel should be. If you're wearing a long peasant skirt, you can wear low ballerina type flats or even low boots. If, however, you're wearing a skirt above knee length, you should probably wear a taller heel.

Sneakers belong with sweat suits, jeans, and some shorts outfits, not with dresses. Flat sandals can be worn with shorts, jeans, or long summery dresses.

When you are shoe shopping, you are faced with a choice: Do you buy what everyone else is wearing or what looks best on you? We hope you'll be able to find shoes that make you comfortable on both counts.

When you are shopping for heels, remember that shoes with ankle straps are generally unflattering unless you have long legs. The strap across the ankle visually makes a horizontal line across the leg, making it appear shorter and stubbier. Try to find light shoes that are comfortable. No matter how glamorous the shoe, if every step in it is an effort, you won't look or feel your best.

For more casual wear, moccasins, ballet slippers, flat boots, and sandals are classic shoe styles that will last forever. But if you are shorter than five feet seven, try to find these styles with a slight heel to look your best.

If you can only afford a few pairs of shoes (and if your feet are still growing, it would be wise to wait a few years before you plan a permanent shoe wardrobe), buy shoes in neutral colors. Tan or brown leather is always in style, and black shoes for winter and white or off-white shoes for summer are also a good bet. Remember, though, that white enlarges and emphasizes, so if you have large feet, go with an off-white or bone color.

One more piece of advice about shoes: flip flops may be cute and fun for summer, but they're the worst things for your feet.

Angie is typing this with her foot in a walking boot—the result of having stepped into a sidewalk crack while wearing flip flops. She had no support for her foot, so she fell and fractured one of those amazing foot bones. She never realized how much she depended on her feet until one of them was out of commission.

Hangnails: A Painful Annoyance

Nearly everyone has known the pain of a hangnail, that tiny piece of skin near the nail that splits painfully away from the cuticle and announces its presence. A hangnail is an inflamed cuticle that has split from the skin, usually as a result of nail-biting or picking at the nail.

To prevent hangnails, keep your fingers and cuticles moisturized with lotion or even olive oil. If the skin is soft and supple, it's less likely to tear and rip off.

If you develop a hangnail, first soak your finger in warm water to soften it, then sterilize a pair of cuticle nippers by dipping them in alcohol. Carefully cut the hangnail off. Apply antiseptic to avoid infection in the area. If the hangnail is already inflamed or infected, see a doctor.

Basic Nail Care

Your nail's worst enemies are water, chemicals, and carelessness. If you have to wash dishes every day, wear gloves. Don't use your nails as a screwdriver or a scraper. And never go out in the freezing cold without gloves.

A manicure is essential for basic nail care. A well-done manicure isn't just "makeup" for the hands, it provides protection for your nails. A weekly manicure is fine; in fact, you should never apply nail polish remover more than once every five days. The chemicals in polish remover are too drying for the nails and can actually weaken them.

Tools for the Perfect Manicure

To begin your manicure, you'll need a few tools you can pick up at any drugstore:

☐ An orangewood stick — for cleaning under the nails and gently pushing back cuticles.

☐ Toenail clippers — a large pair, designed to cut straight across for toenails, and a small pair for trimming extra long

65

fingernails.

☐   Emery boards — use the tan emery boards for your toenails, but for your fingers, use the black ones for shaping and a blue or pink buffing disc or a smoothie (an emery-board look-alike with a foam core, without sandpaper).

☐   Nail polish remover — use an oily or non-acetone formula if your nails tend to be dry or brittle.

☐   Nail polishes — any kind will do. There's no reason to buy expensive ones.

☐   Cuticle softener—not cuticle remover. Your fingers need cuticles to seal out dirt and bacteria. Baby oil works well as a cuticle softener, and prevents tears and hangnails.

☐   Liquid fiber-wrap base coat — if your nails are peeling or weak, these base coats with fibers can repair small breaks.

☐   A base coat and top coat — these help prevent nail staining and keep the color of the nail enamel true. A top coat also helps your nail enamel resist chipping and makes your nails stronger.

The Perfect Manicure

Begin your manicure by removing your old polish with a cotton ball. Wet the cotton ball with nail polish remover and hold it on your nail for a few seconds to soften the old coat. Then wipe forward, *away* from the cuticle. If your nails have been stained by the old polish, rub a fresh lemon across your nails.

Next, shape your nails. With a fine-grained emery board held at a forty-five degree angle to the nail, begin to gently file in one direction only. Don't saw back and forth, and avoid the fragile corners of your nails. Smooth any rough edges with a buffing disc. To test the smoothness of your nails, run them across an old pair of pantyhose and see if they catch.

What shape should your nails be? The most natural shape for nails would result if you followed the shape of your nail base, which could be round, square, pointed, or oval. Don't just file the edges of your nails, but try to make the shape of the free edge mirror the shape of your nail base.

If you have short hands and short fingers, you might find that your best look is oval nails, which will seem to lengthen your fingers. If your nails have a rounded base, shape your nails gently into a soft square on the free edge with slightly rounded corners. Very narrow nails need a soft square look. Keep in mind that pointed nails look dreadful on everyone.

What length should your nails be? Try to overcome the feeling that long is good and longer is better. "Dragon lady" nails are out of style and tend to look artificial and tacky. Today *anyone* can glue on two-inch nails!

There are three basic lengths you should consider. *Short* nails extend to the tip of the finger. The free edge of *average length* nails extends past the finger tip one-fourth the length of the nail plate. The free edge of *long nails* extends past the finger tip one-third to one-half the length of the nail plate. Anything that doubles the length of the nail plate is really too long.

If you need help determining the best length for you, Elisa Ferri offers the following quiz:

1.   Do your nails turn up or down at the ends? If so, keep your nails short.

2.   Do you do a lot of swimming? Ice skating? Skiing? Working at the computer? Playing piano? If so, avoid long nails.

3.   Are your hands small in proportion to your body size? If so, longer nails will be more flattering.

4.   Are your hands large in proportion to your body size? If so, keep your nails at average length.

5.   Are your fingers thick and your hands large? Try nails slightly longer than average length.[1]

After shaping your nails, soften your cuticles. Apply the cuticle softener around the cuticles, then soak your dominant hand in warm soapy water for five minutes. You may want to brush your nails with a soft brush or an old toothbrush.

Remove your hand and gently push back the cuticles with the flat end of an orangewood stick, being careful not to scratch the nail plate. Then use the orangewood stick to clean under the nail. Do not cut your cuticles. Remove any hangnails with a pair of sterile cuticle nippers with a short snipping and pulling motion. Repeat the process with the other hand.

If you prefer not to polish your nails, buff them. Apply a small dab of paste polish to each nail with your fingertip. Buff your nails with a buffer, stroking from the base to the edge or from side to side until your nails are smooth and glossy.

Before you apply nail polish, clean up your area and put away your equipment except for an orangewood stick, your nail polish remover, and your nail enamel, base coat, and top coat. Place the orangewood stick in the bottle of nail polish remover for quick clean ups of the polish which may end up on the skin outside your nail.

Now that you're ready to polish, begin with a base coat. If you have problem nails that chip or peel, use a base coat of liquid fiber wrap. Apply one coat horizontally, from side to side, and let it dry. Then apply another coat vertically, from the nail base to the free edge. Allow this coat five minutes to dry.

Select your nail enamel. When polishing, polish your dominant hand first, beginning with the little finger and working toward your thumb. As you polish, paint the tips of the nails with quick strokes, then in three sweeping strokes, paint from the nail base to the edge, the center first, then the two sides. Wipe off any excess polish with the orangewood stick. Allow the polish to dry for two minutes, then repeat. Allow the polish to dry five minutes before applying the top coat.

If your nail polish "bubbles" as you apply it, it's likely that you're using old polish, are sitting in a draft, or have oil on your hands. If you smudge your polish during the manicure, put a drop of nail polish remover on the meaty portion of your thumb and rub it lightly over the smudge until it is smooth, then reapply the polish.

Apply a clear top coat, and allow it to dry for ten minutes. You might want to try some of the new nail enamels that contain fast-evaporating ingredients such as Sally Hansen Dries Instantly Protective Top Coat, which dries in less than thirty seconds.

Whatever enamels you choose, after a good manicure your nails will be beautiful, strong, and protected.

Nail Color

What color should you wear on your nails? The huge range of colors available tends to be overwhelming, so if you narrow your selections to certain shades, you'll be more likely to choose colors that really flatter you. You should try to find colors that look good with your skin tone.

Whatever colors you choose, don't (please!) fall prey to fads such as black polish, stripes, decals, etc. Such things are totally trendy, and while they may be fun for a while, they're pretty bizarre and only draw attention to your nails — not to *you*.

Color tips:

☐   If you wear "warm" colors on your nails, try to wear "warm" clothing colors, too. You'll look really together!

☐   If you have active hands, clear and sheer colors don't show chips as easily as dark colors.

☐   If you've worn one color all week and want a change for the weekend, put a top coat of dark or bright polish over your nails for a quick change before the next manicure.

☐   Toenails don't have to be the same color as your fingers; in fact, toenails often need a deeper color to show up in sandals. But make sure the colors of your toes and fingers don't clash.

French Manicure

The French Manicure is increasingly popular and versatile, and you can give yourself one at home. You'll need a sheer nude or beige polish and a white, ivory, or pale pink polish.

To give yourself a French manicure, follow our "how to manicure" steps we've already given you. When you are ready to polish, use a watercolor or eyeliner brush to apply the white, ivory, or pale pink polish to the *edge only* of each nail (where your nail is naturally white). Allow the polish to dry for three minutes.

Now, over the entire nail, apply a coat of sheer nude beige, sheer pink, or any other transparent color. Let it dry for five minutes, then repeat with another coat of sheer polish. That's it. You've now got a chic French manicure. The best thing about a French manicure is that it looks natural, your nails are protected, and chips hardly show at all. It's a very professional, polished look.

Nail Biting

If you bite your nails, don't feel like you're all alone. When Princess Diana was first engaged to Prince Charles, one of the most striking things about her official portraits was that this elegant and beautiful young woman was obviously a nail-biter. We've noticed in later photos that while she still has neat and tidy nails, they're not as ragged as they used to be.

Angie used to bite her nails, too. During her first year of college she taught organ lessons and was literally embarrassed out of the habit when one of her organ students, an older woman, lifted her hand and asked, "Why do you bite your nails? You're a beautiful girl, and you have nothing to be nervous about!"

That did it for Angie. She didn't bite her nails because she was nervous; it was only a bad habit. But from that day forward she decided she'd take pride in her nails, and she licked (sorry, bad pun) the nail-biting habit.

If you'd like to stop biting your nails, you can break the habit too. First, you should know that nail biting not only is embarrassing, but it takes bacteria from your busy fingers and transfers them to your mouth. Even if you don't actually *bite* your nails, but just pick at them, you'll be prone to hangnails and infections because our hands are in contact with all sorts of bacteria.

To kick the habit, visit your drug store or beauty supply shop and spend a little money to stress your commitment to your nails. For our simple program, you'll need to purchase a cuticle softener, a nail buffing disc, and clear nail polish. Then set aside a regular time each week to follow this routine:

1.   First apply a cuticle softener to your cuticles and give your hands a fifteen-minute oil and water soak to soften your extra-tough cuticles.

2.   Gently push your cuticles back. If they are very overgrown or ragged at first, have a professional manicurist trim them.

3.   Use a buffing disc to file over any rough edges on the top of your nail and at the free edge. Keep the buffing disc with you (in your purse, maybe?) at all times so if you feel a rough edge on your nails, you can smooth it immediately instead of worrying with it until you've ripped away another nail.

4.   Moisturize your nails and cuticles with a good hand cream or petroleum jelly.

5.   Give yourself a full manicure every three or four days for two months to eliminate all rough edges as they grow out.

6.   Apply clear nail polish. This step is very important If you're tempted to put your hands in your mouth, bad-tasting nail polish is also available at your drug store.

Artificial Nails

Some women absolutely love artificial nails. Acrylic nails, professionally applied, look good, don't chip, and last for up to two weeks. But they require careful maintenance, can be expensive, and can cause problems.

If you're interested in a set of acrylic sculptured nails, make an appointment at a *clean* salon. Plan to spend one hour and between forty and one hundred dollars for a full set of nails. You can also count on weekly or biweekly appointments for fill-ins that will cost between fifteen and fifty dollars. This maintenance is important to prevent moisture and dirt from becoming trapped under the nail and resulting in infection and/or fungus growth. Remember, acrylic nails are not indestructible: They may loosen after long soaks in the tub or pool or rubs with creams or oils.

There are several different methods of nail application. Some salons apply tips first, others insert a nail form under the existing nail's free edge and "build" a new nail out from the real nail.

Before you decide to splurge on sculptured nails, you should know two things: First, in rare situations the real nail can separate from the nail bed because portions of the nail plate adhere to the false nail. Second, if you decide that acrylic nails are not for you after a month or so of wearing them, it may take up to a year for your own nails to grow out to their normal strength.

Angie got a set of acrylic nails once, and after a few months she ripped them off and decided to let her own nails grow out. But when she removed the false nails, slivers from the nail plate of her own nails came off as well. Her nails had already been weakened because the manicurist "roughed up" their surfaces so the acrylic would have a rough surface to cling to. Nearly a year passed before Angie's nails were back to their normal strength and thickness. But, she admits, the false nails were fun while they lasted. You have to decide for yourself whether you have the time and money to invest in the care and upkeep of acrylic nails.

Laura's Hand Helpers

✓ Use rubber gloves when doing dishes, washing the car, etc. Rub baby oil on your hands before you put on the gloves and you'll be moisturizing your hands while you do your chores!

☐ Rub petroleum jelly on your hands and cover them with a pair of gloves before bed. If your hands get dry and rough in winter, this will keep them springtime soft!

☐ You can remove ink and other stains from your hands and fingers by rubbing them with a cut lemon.

☐ Give your nails a chance to breathe by taking off the old polish at night and waiting until morning to reapply new polish and complete your manicure.

☐ Make it a habit to use hand cream after washing your hands. Keep a pump dispenser of moisturizing cream by the kitchen and bathroom sinks.

☐ Dark shades of nail polish call attention to your nails. If your nails are short or ragged, use lighter, more natural shades.

Remember, you can be your best from your head to your toes.

7
YOUR PASSION FOR FASHION

Before going to early morning modeling shoots, model Megan follows beauty advice from her grandmother:

> Puffy morning eyes are never welcome, especially in this business. My grandmother's advice still stands-apply wet, cold tea bags to your eyes. It really works!

Whether you're going to a modeling shoot or to school, your eyes should look good — and so should your clothes. Your choice is to wear clothes that help you look your best or settle for any old thing you pull out of the closet. We want you to be your best.

Understand Your Growing Body

At puberty, when your hormones signal that it's time to mature, your breasts, hips, and pubic hair begin to grow. In adolescence your body loses the straight lines of childhood and becomes more womanly and rounded.

When you begin to develop a woman's body, don't assume that you're getting too heavy or that you need to go on a diet. Give your body some time to adjust to the changes. If you are eating good food and staying active, you should find that your maturing body is a perfect fit for you!

Many girls don't really know what shape or size their bodies are. In one study, a researcher showed women pictures of bodies in

73

different sizes and asked them to choose the pictures that showed what their bodies looked like. Women consistently chose pictures larger than they really were.[1]

We all grew up with Barbie dolls. If we zapped a Barbie doll with an enlarging gun and made her life size, her measurements would be 36-20-32. Impossible to achieve, at least not without breast implants and a corset. But that is the doll we all grew up with, a plastic, stiff-armed smiling doll with three ounces of hair and tiny, high-heeled feet.

In many homes today, Barbie has been replaced by the "Happy to Be Me" doll, like Barbie in nearly every way but body shape. The Happy doll's measurements in life-size would be 36-27-38, which is much more realistic for a fully developed girl.

Understand Your Body Line

Every body is different, and chances are you're not just like your best friend. But bodies do fall into different categories, and if you understand your basic body type, you'll be able to choose fashions that look best on you.

One of the best ways to define your body type is by studying your shadow. Find an empty wall in your house and stand in your underwear with a lamp directly behind you.

Study your shadow carefully. Are your hips wider than your bustline? Is your waistline narrow or naturally thick? Do your legs seem long or short in comparison to your torso?

Endomorphs are people with large frames, what people usually call "big bones." If you're an endomorph, your thighs, buttocks, and breasts may be round and full. Your hips will be slightly wider than your shoulders. Mae West was an endomorph.

Ectomorphs are usually tall and thin, with small, flat hips the same width as their shoulders. The entire silhouette will appear to be rectangular, and your arms and legs may seem long in relation to your torso. Princess Diana was an ectomorph.

Mesomorphs are medium bodies with curved hips, shaped waists, and a full bustline. The silhouette is softer and more curved, and the shoulders are usually wider than the hips. Elizabeth Taylor was a mesomorph.

Learning to be your beautiful best means coming to terms with the basic body shape you've inherited from your parents. While you may be able to change the size of your body through exercise and/or diet, you won't be able to change its basic shape. You'll have to make the best of it, just like you learn to cope with curly or straight hair. But no matter what kind of "morph" you are, you can make yourself beautiful!

Proportion in Fashion

It's important to understand proportion if you want to dress to be your best. There's a simple guiding rule behind proportion: If you make one part of your body look longer, another part will look smaller. For instance, if you have long legs and wear high-waisted slacks with a four-inch belt, your torso will look even shorter than it usually is. If you have short legs and wear a long jacket over slacks, your torso will look longer and your legs shorter. By combining your clothes more carefully, you can help your body look more balanced.

Texture and color also help to balance an outfit. Obviously, a bulky cable knit sweater that ends at your hips will make you look hip-heavy. But if you wear the sweater with navy pants and a navy scarf at your neckline, the viewer's eye will be drawn up to the splash of color at your neck, not at the bulk around your waist and hips.

Find Your Thin Lines

If you want to wear clothes that make you look slimmer or fuller, the key is simple: *learn to look for lines in clothing.* Your outfit may not have a stripe on it, but it definitely has lines.

Where's the clothing line in an outfit that consists of white shorts and a blue, tucked-in T-shirt? At the waistline. The two colors come together in a horizontal line at the waist. Where's the line if you wear the T-shirt out? Probably at the hips, where the hem falls.

Imagine a solid green woman's dress that buttons down the center front from neck to hem. Where's the clothing line? It's a vertical line straight down the middle. Imagine the same dress in a green stripe—where's the clothing line? The buttons will fade to invisibility in all those stripes, and the line (lines, actually) will be in whatever direction the stripes are going. If you want to look slimmer, wear clothing with long, diagonal lines or vertical lines that run from top to bottom. Horizontal lines will make you look thicker.

Vertical lines are found in longer jackets in suits and dresses. Vertical patterns in printed fabrics will give the same illusion, but if you want to create a slimming effect, avoid polka dots, geometric, or checkered plaids. If you're wearing an outfit without vertical lines, you can create one by wearing a long strand of beads, a long chain, scarf, or tie.

The Principles of Dressing Thin

Let's examine some specific areas and ways to "dress thin." Even if you're the perfect weight, you may wish to disguise certain characteristics of your body shape. No one wants to look too bulky.

If you have wide hips, wear lighter colors on top and a splash of color at your neckline to take the viewer's eye upward.

Pleated skirts with a pleat that begins *below* the hips would be very slimming for you. They are known as "stitched down pleats" because the pleats are stitched down to the hipline. Avoid pleats and gathers at the waistline if you want to look thinner in the hip area. Wrap skirts are also slimming, but keep skirts simple.

Pants for the full-hipped woman should also be simple. Avoid pants that are gathered or pleated at the waistline as well as tight pants with skinny legs and tight ankles. Those will make your hips seem even wider by comparison.

If you're concerned about a large or heavy bustline, remember to wear darker colors on top. The best camouflage for a heavy bustline is clothing. Remember that bright colors emphasize, deeper colors disguise. If you're larger at the bustline than at the hips, avoid clingy fabrics and tight fits and opt for jackets whenever possible (just avoid jackets with a pinched-in waist— they're for smaller girls who want to emphasize the bustline).

In general, you can "dress thin" by avoiding bulky fabrics and horizontal lines *anywhere*. Look for slimming up and down lines. Simple V-necklines and A-line dresses are wonderful for dressing thin because they draw attention to your face, but if you have a heavy bust, avoid V-necks with huge ruffles. Also avoid round necklines, unless you wear a long chain or long necklace. Square necklines are fine, but they're even better if you add a scarf, ribbons, a vest, or a long chain to create a slimming horizontal line.

If you want to dress thin, avoid heavily gathered sleeves that add bulk to your silhouette. Tailored long sleeves are fine, but most short sleeves end just above your elbow in a mini-horizontal line. To help rid yourself of this non-slimming line, roll your sleeve up once. If your arms are heavy, avoid three-quarter length sleeves and sleeveless dresses and blouses.

If you're self-conscious about being large, you may shudder at the thought of exposing your waistband, but waistbands define the waist and actually slim your silhouette as long as they are not too tight. A bulging tummy under a too-tight waistband is not a slim picture. Avoid wide waistbands and belts unless you're very long-waisted. Remember, the longer look is the slimmer look.

Some women think that by wearing clothes that are too small, they are dressing thin, but the opposite is true. It is better to wear a well-fitting size fourteen than to squeeze yourself into a too-tight ten and have the material bunch and pucker. Women who dress "thin" avoid bulky or thick fabrics and tight, bright belts. Neutral colors are best.

Big Can Be Beautiful

"Some of the prettiest girls in the modeling business are large-size models," says Laura. If you wear a large size, don't think you're resigned to wearing tent dresses and tops. Lillian Russell and Mae West were always known for their beauty, but neither was a small woman. Big can be beautiful as long as you don't try to squeeze yourself into clothes that are too small.

If you are big-boned or carry extra pounds, don't put off buying nice clothes. "I'll wait until I lose some weight," you may think. "Then I'll really look good."

The time to be your best is *now*. Don't put it off. Don't decide not to care about yourself until you're five or ten or twenty pounds lighter. You are the same person you will be no matter what your weight, and you need to care about yourself *now*. If you're large, look for and wear clothes that are comfortable, in good taste, and fit well. "Comfortable" does not mean ugly. We all have cast-off clothing at home that really belongs in the rag bag, but we keep them around because they're "comfortable." Go ahead and throw out those uglies!

Many larger girls have a tendency to hide themselves in clothes that are too big. Wearing humongous clothes won't make you any smaller, but it will make you *look* larger. You don't have to wear tent dresses and huge overblouses. You don't have to stick to dark clothing. And you shouldn't pretend to be invisible.

You can be proud of yourself just the way you are. If today you've made a decision to be the best you can be, you're already better than you were yesterday. You're on the road to beauty, and you can carry yourself with confidence, so don't hide under dark, baggy tent dresses.

Petite Problems

Some girls are so petite, they'd give anything to gain ten pounds or grow two inches. According to the National Center for Health Statistics, 55 percent of American women are five feet, four inches or shorter. Fortunately for these women, many manufacturers offer clothing in petite sizes.

If you are petite, remember that vertical lines lengthen. Wear clothing with vertical lines or stripes and prepare to visually grow. Avoid long tunics and tops; short jackets will make your legs appear longer.

If you're petite, you can wear horizontal lines, large prints, plaids, and heavy fabrics. If you are small-busted, you can enhance your figure by wearing lots of ruffles, gathers, yokes, tucks, and blouson styles. Avoid the bare look that exposes your arms and narrow shoulders, and you should also avoid skin-hugging, clingy fabrics.

Stringbeans

Laura knows what it's like to be made fun of because you're tall and thin. "I hated it. I was taller than all the boys," she says. "But now I wouldn't trade my height for anything."

If you're five feet seven or taller, pants are usually too short, sleeves hit your arm above the wrist bone, and wearing one-piece rompers and jumpsuits is a physical impossibility!

If you are tall, wear longer tops and jackets. You will be able to successfully wear many high-fashion designs, since these are designed for tall women. If you're long-waisted, wide belts will accent your waistline and de-emphasize your longer torso.

Several stores and catalogs like L.L. Bean and Lands End carry some pants in long or tall sizes and may even hem them to your specifications. Being tall isn't a problem for Laura she just orders her dress pants from Lands End. Spiegel and J.C. Penney also offer a selection of dresses, blouses, and pants in tall sizes.

Fashion Begins Underneath

It's impossible to be well-dressed if you're not well dressed down to the skin. Mothers across America are famous for saying, "Wear good underwear--you might end up in the hospital!" but there's more than one reason to choose underwear that looks good and fits well.

Bras are important because the female breast has no muscle tissue. You can't exercise your way to firmer breasts. The pectoral muscles do lie under the breasts and firm pecs can make your breasts appear larger, but these muscles have little to do with the breasts themselves.

Your breasts are composed of fibrous, connective, and fatty tissues. They will grow as you do, and there are no exercises or pills or devices that will make them grow faster or bigger. You've got what you've got, and there's little anyone but a plastic surgeon can do about it. But the right bra can make a tremendous difference in how you look.

Anyone larger than an A-cup size needs to wear a bra every day. Don't know your cup size? Try the pencil test: Put a pencil under your breast, horizontal to the floor. If it falls, you don't need a bra. If it doesn't fall, going braless might damage the tender tissue of your breasts.

Before you shop for a bra, measure your rib cage immediately under your breasts with a tape measure and add five inches. If the result is an odd number, add one. That number is the band size. To find your cup size, measure again, this time holding the tape measure over the fullest part of your bust. If this measurement is one inch larger than the first measurement, you are an A cup; two inches, a B cup; three inches, a C cup; four inches, a D cup; five inches, a DD cup.

But even this rule of measurement is not set in stone. Bras are constructed differently, and the only way to make sure the bra will fit properly is to try it on. When trying on a bra, bend over at the waist and let your breasts fall comfortably into the cups. Make sure the bra is not too loose, or it will not support you properly. If it is too tight, the straps will dig into your shoulders and the elastic around your rib cage may inhibit your breathing.

There are bras for every type of lifestyle, clothing, and budget Take an afternoon to visit the lingerie department of a department store and you'll see that bras come in plunge, décolleté, halter, strapless, long-line, underwire, padded, and soft-cup styles.

Sports bras are the most supportive bras of all, and they are a must if you are active. Sports bras should be made of absorbent cotton and mostly non-elastic so they will stand up under many machine washings.

When purchasing a bra, keep two things in mind: Colored bras show through light-colored tops, and if you're cold, nervous, or excited, your nipples may show through a thin bra and cause you embarrassment. A bra is a foundation garment. Its purpose is to make the most of what you have, not to call attention to itself or to your "endowments." For these reasons, you may wish to buy white or off-white bras, and unless you want to wear a heavily padded bra to build up your figure, try one with a soft cup. Soft cup bras are lightly padded and prevent embarrassing show-through. Flesh-colored bras won't show through sheer blouses like a white bra.

Proper fit is also important for panties. Whether you wear high-cut briefs, bikini panties, or those with tummy control, make sure the panties are not too tight. Check in the mirror at the end of your day—does your underwear leave red lines along your waist or hips, under your breasts, or at the top of your thighs? If so, you need a larger size. Wearing underwear that is too small doesn't make you look smaller, it only adds and accentuates bulges under your clothes.

One final tip about underwear: Always, but particularly in the summer, wear cotton panties or at least panties with a cotton crotch. Cotton "breathes," therefore it is more healthful and may prevent recurrent yeast infections.

The Suit That Suits You

The creator of the comic strip "Cathy" has a field day with the nightmare of searching for a bathing suit. If a bathing suit looks good, it may not be fashionable, or maybe it's not modest. If you like it, your mother may hate it. If your mom likes it, you wouldn't be caught dead in it. Or maybe you won't be caught dead in any bathing suit because you think you're too (choose one!) big, flat, fat, or skinny.

Believe it or not, shopping for a bathing suit has become easier. There are more suits available these days, and one of them can help you look good.

If you're self-conscious about small breasts, look for bathing suit styles that are gathered, frilled, or shirred at the top or that have stripes or patterns at the bust line. Velvet would be a good fabric for you because it's bulky. Look for a bathing suit with padding. (They even have a new one with inflatable cups, but that's going a bit too far, don't you think?)

If you are self-conscious about large breasts, look for bathing suits in darker colors that feature underwire or built-in bras. Choose straps that cross in back for better support. If you have a thick waistline, a V-neck suit (or a suit with a V anywhere on the front) will add length and slimness to your torso. A belted suit is ideal for you. Also look for tank suits with diagonals or racing stripes down the sides. Off-the-shoulder styles will make your waist seem tiny.

If you have an ample fanny, avoid suits with high cut legs. Look for one-piece suits with buttons and bows on top. Small patterns are best on patterned suits, or wear two-toned suits with the darker color on the bottom. To balance your shoulders with wide hips, choose a suit with inset shoulder straps. Diagonal stripes will draw attention away from your body, and never, ever wear horizontal stripes.

If you have short legs and a long torso, horizontal or wild prints are for you. Avoid diagonal or vertical stripes, which will only accent your long torso. High-cut legs are good for you, since they lengthen the leg area.

If you wish to disguise a bulging tummy, find a bathing suit with strong diagonal stripes or one of the front-wrap suits. If you choose to wear a two-piece bathing suit, wear one that covers your belly button with elastic. The basic black tank suit is a good choice for you.

Today's swimsuit manufacturers are now selling "slim suits" that actually reduce your waistline. The Miraclesuit claims to make its wearers look ten pounds thinner because it's constructed of a new fabric with three times as much Lycra spandex as the average swimsuit — that's supposed to be three times the holding power. The Slim Suit (sold at J.C. Penney and other stores) features an inner lining that acts as a body girdle. It is guaranteed to take an inch or more off the average waistline.

The Land's End catalog offers a new line of swimwear called "Kindest Cut" that features modest necklines, sensible seat coverage and is sized to fit both long and short torsos.[2]

There have never been so many suits from which you can choose. Whether you want an old-fashioned look or the latest thing, there's a bathing suit that will fit both your body and your personality. But remember, showing everything on the beach is uncool. You may draw attention, but it won't be the right kind!

Buying Tips for Shopping Trips

You're in the store salivating over the most *gorgeous* $100 dress. It'd be perfect for the special night you have planned, and you have saved all summer's babysitting money so you have the money. Should you buy the dress?

Maybe. (Bet you thought we were going to say no!) If you can wear the dress more than twice, in fact, if you can wear it several times, it may be a good buy.

But if an article of clothing doesn't fit right, itches, needs pinning, is the wrong color, isn't comfortable, is stained or torn, or needs altering, it's *not* a bargain. The same principle is true for jewelry, shoes, and purses.

When trying on shirts or blouses, look in the mirror to check the fit. Are there gaps between the buttons? If there are, the shirt is too tight or the buttons are spaced incorrectly. Now bend forward from your waistline and look at your back in the mirror. Does any skin show? If so, the shirt is too short.

If you're trying on a skirt or pants, make sure you can insert your two thumbs at the waistline. Hold in your tummy and pinch the waistband. You should be able to gather at least one inch of fabric, and not more than two inches.

Don't shop when you're depressed, don't shop in a crisis, and don't buy something just because it's 50 percent off. In order for an article of clothing to be a good addition to your wardrobe, it should match something you already have and you should be able to wear it more than four times.

If you're shopping for a dress, wear a dress while shopping. You'll have a better idea of how the dress will look. It's always a little confusing to try on a nice dress when your jeans are gathered around your ankles and the toes of your sneakers are peeping out. You might want to throw an extra pair of dress shoes in your bag so you'll have a better idea of the finished outfit while you're still in the dressing room.

You'll have the best success shopping if you begin planning your wardrobe at the beginning of the season. For instance, fall clothing begins arriving in the stores in August, and most stores hold decent pre-season sales to get their new merchandise moving. You'll have the best selection if you shop early. If you wait until February you may not have a good selection, but you'll have clearance prices.

As you shop, learn to tell the difference between a "classic" item and something that is faddish. Classic clothes like jeans, knit shirts, tennis shoes, and simple skirts have been and will be around forever. Faddish shoes (platform or "Jelly" shoes, miniskirts) usually spring onto the scene and disappear quietly after making a big splash. Don't spend your hard-earned money on faddish clothes. If something is fun and inexpensive, fine, enjoy it for a season. But don't invest your life in it.

Memorize the Tacky Twelve

Imagine Sylvia descending the stairs to host her first party. You are standing at the bottom of the stairs, looking up at your friend. Sylvia's hair is smooth and golden, falling neatly into place and swaying gently as she steps gracefully down the stairs. She's wearing a sleeveless white wrap dress that flatters her willowy form. A single elegant gold bracelet shines lightly on her wrist. Her legs are smooth and long, but your eye stops and stares at her feet. Peeping from her beach sandals, Sylvia's bright red toenail polish is chipped and rough, and there's an unmistakable smudge of black dirt across her hairy big toe.

How tacky. This illustration serves to remind us that one little thing can absolutely ruin an elegant and beautiful appearance. Certain things offset the image of beauty, and if you memorize our "Tacky Twelve" list and avoid them, you'll be on your way to *always* looking great.

1.   Tacky is a missing button. Don't wear a shirt, dress, or blouse with a missing button.
2.   Tacky is noisy, jangling jewelry. People will be so annoyed by the noise you make, they'll forget about your pleasing appearance. Keep your favorite charm bracelet in a drawer.
3.   Tacky is having your bra or slip strap show from under your clothes. Yes, really.

4. Tacky is panty lines that show through a tight skirt or pants.

5. Tacky is dirty clothes or a dragging hem.

6. Tacky is shoes that need repair.

7. Tacky is shoes that clack as you walk.

8. Tacky is any kind of hose with runs. Tackier is hose with runs and bright red gobs of fingernail polish to stop the runs.

9. Tacky is wearing reinforced toe panty hose with sandals.

10. Tacky is super-long fingernails.

11. Tacky is an elegant dress or skirt with a revealing slit, and tackier still is a slip showing through the slit.

12. Tacky is an untidy person, marked by lack of style, good taste, or by cheap showiness. (We thank *Webster's Dictionary* for this last definition.)

Is there hope for the terribly tacky? Sure there is. Just clean up your act and resolve that you will be tacky no more. Of course we've all had tacky days. No one can help occasionally getting a run in a pair of panty hose, and not many women leave home every day with a spare pair. But we can all memorize the list and do our best to avoid the Tacky Twelve.

Confidence Boosters

If you don't have many clothes or feel terribly unfashionable, you can still be confident in your appearance by taking care of what you do have.

Too often we get into a clothing rut, always grabbing whatever is convenient. If you'll get into the habit of always returning your clothing to the closet in a certain place, you'll get more and better wear from the clothes you have. For instance, the next time you need a pair of pants, choose a pair from the *left* side of the pants section in your closet. After you've worn and washed the pants, return them to the *right* side of the pants section. The pair of pants will gradually slide down to the left, but not before you've worn most of the other pants in your closet. You'll be rotating your clothing evenly and not wearing the same things over and over. Everyone will marvel at the variety of your wardrobe!

Sweaters and sweat suits can be stored in a drawer or on a shelf, but don't store them in plastic or plastic bags. Clothing needs to breathe. When you put clothes that have been dry cleaned back into your closet, carefully snip all but six inches of the cleaner's plastic bag away. You'll be left with a six-inch "dust cover" to protect the top of your clothing, and the material will still be able to breathe.

If your closet is musty and humid, fill a coffee can with charcoal briquettes, punch holes in the plastic lid, and keep the can on the floor of the closet. The charcoal will absorb humidity. If your closet has a bad smell, buy a bar of scented deodorant soap, unwrap it, and place it on the shelf in your closet for springtime freshness.

Quick Tips to Becoming a Stylish Standout

Belts are a great fashion accessory because they draw the viewer's eye to your waist. Avoid wide belts if your waistline is thick.

Have an extra pierced earring because you lost its mate? Use it as a tiny pin to hold a scarf in place around your neck. Lose the back of your pierced earring at school? Break the eraser off a pencil and use it to hold your earring in place for the rest of the day.

Dress up a plain outfit with lace. Wear lacy stockings, insert a lace hankie in your pocket, or wear a lacy camisole under a jacket. Nothing looks as feminine as lace!

Have a pretty pin and no place to wear it? Hang it on a necklace that's choker length. Or wear it on your shoulder, to draw the viewer's eye upward. Or place it on a grosgrain ribbon (measure your neck plus six inches) and wear it as a pretty choker. Tired of wearing scarves around your neck? Twist two long scarves together and wear them as a colorful belt. Tie a scarf to your shoulder bag for a splash of color. Or wear a scarf on the outside collar of your coat to match your winter hat.

Choose a stocking color that is one shade lighter than your shoes unless you want your stockings to make a fashion statement.

Dress Says So Much

We've talked about how to make yourself look good, how to flatter your figure, organize your closet, and buy the clothes you add to your wardrobe. Before we leave this chapter, though, we want to ask you one question: Why do you dress the way you do? What do you want your clothes to say to others?

We've all had the experience of picking up a dress or blouse and saying, "This looks just like Aunt Jenny." (Okay, maybe not Aunt Jenny, but you know what we mean.) Your clothes say a lot about you, and that image is so strong that sometimes just seeing a dress or shirt can remind people of you.

What does your typical look say to the world who's watching you? Does it say, "I don't really care what I look like" or "Hey, I'm okay because I look like everybody else"? You can be an individual, and your dress should echo the high standards in your life.

Angie went to high school in the days of the mini-skirt and remembers reading in fashion magazines that "midis" were coming into style. (For those of you who didn't grow up in the '70s, midis were long skirts that came to mid-calf.) No one at Angie's school had worn one yet, but Angie was tired of having to be careful every time she sat down or leaned over to pick something up. Mini-skirts were not the easiest things to move around in!

Anyway, Angie went home from school one day, visited the fabric store, and whipped up two mid-calf length skirts. She wore them to school and never felt more comfortable in her life. It didn't matter that everyone else stared — she was on the cutting edge of fashion, she knew it, and she could finally move freely!

So don't be afraid to try something that's different. As long as the innovation will help you look your best, as long as it is modest and practical, go for it!

Is Modesty Out of Style?

What about modesty? What is it, and should you be concerned about it? Modesty, as defined by *Webster's,* is "propriety [doing what is proper] in dress, speech, and conduct." According to Webster, modest dress is proper dress. What is proper in one place might not be proper somewhere else.

You can wear a one-piece bathing suit on the beach and be entirely modest and proper. Wearing the same bathing suit in the grocery store is neither. Laura has found that you can wear a shorter skirt in New York City, the fashion capitol of the world, and be entirely modest and proper. Wearing the same shorter skirt in Kansas City may be neither.

Modesty is also concerned with being considerate of others. Most men will frankly tell you that they are physically stimulated by sight, and most men are stimulated by the sight of breasts, legs, and thighs. Therefore, if you wear clothing that reveals or hints at exposing your breasts or thighs, you're waving a red flag to the average man whether you intend to or not.

You don't have to go through life in clothes buttoned up to your neck and skirts down to your ankles, but you should use common sense when you dress. You don't have to dress to hide your figure. Most fashions today show your figure to some degree, and it's okay to present a trim and shapely appearance. But don't wear shorts so short that your buttocks are exposed when you bend over. Don't wear pants so tight that your panty lines show through. Don't wear see-through blouses that leave nothing to the imagination. If you ever have a doubt about whether or not an outfit is modest, don't ask your mom or your best friend. Ask your father or your brother.

The entire world, including many fashion magazine ads, would have you think that to look good you have to look hot, sizzlingly sexy. That's just not true. If a guy looks your way only because you look sexy, he's not seeing the real you at all. He's only seeing the shell, and who wants a relationship based on that? Your dress doesn't have to appeal to the lust market. Instead, dress to look your beautiful best.

Laura says, "Modesty is a fine line, and even I have trouble with that sometimes. I think it boils down to this: Are you dressing to be in style or to get attention and be sexy? There have been times I tried on a stylish dress that I thought was too sexy, so I didn't buy it. I don't like being stared at by men in the subway or on the street. The most important thing is to find what suits you and what shows you at your best without trying to draw attention to yourself.

"There are a lot of fashions that make women look beautiful without making them look sexy. I sometimes worry about young girls now, though, because there's a big lust market out there. But if you're dressing to attract someone to you physically, then you're asking for a superficial — and dangerous—relationship. There's always going to be somebody to outdo you, some girl that's prettier or sexier.

"But we don't find our freedom and ultimate security in how we look. You can say, 'This is who I am, and I don't need to compete, or buy this or that to be accepted.'"

Perhaps we can say it best by saying it bluntly: If your dress advertises your body like goods for sale, don't be surprised if you're treated like a prostitute. To be treated with the respect you deserve, dress like a lady.

8
FITNESS FUN

Jordan, another model friend of Laura's, knows that exercise is important for health and beauty:

> Our bodies are a little like cars, you know? You can't keep them in the garage for months and then expect to win a long-distance race. God designed our bodies to get us through a lifetime of living, but we've got to keep them in good running order.

Angie's Story

Between 1987 and 1990, I joined two exercise groups and a spa, purchased two exercise videos, two exercise books, three aerobic exercise albums, two sets of dumbbells, and thirteen books on eating for fitness. Between 1987 and 1990, I actually exercised ten times.

I supported every woman's right to don athletic shoes and sweat. I knew that women feel better after exercising. They eat less, burn more calories, reduce their chances for osteoporosis (hunched backs) in old age, have more energy, and sleep better at night. Trouble was, I just couldn't get motivated to exercise myself.

Every now and then, usually after watching the Olympics or a Rocky movie, I'd be overcome by a wave of guilt. "Okay, body," I'd mutter, looking down at legs that used to climb mountains and march in the band, "time to get to it!" But after a full day of my normal routine, I'd rather crash into the TV chair with a plate of

Little Debbies than sweat to the oldies with Richard Simmons.

Once, after watching *The Turning Point* with Mikhail Baryshnikov, I gathered my gumption and signed up for ballet classes. I was the only adult woman in a room of eight-year-olds. After one lesson, the thrill was gone.

But one day I made a simple decision to get off my duff and exercise, thrill or no thrill. I got up, ate my breakfast, did thirty minutes of exercises with an eager lady on television, showered, and sat down at my desk to work. I follow the same routine every weekday now, without thought or hesitation. And I do sleep better, feel better, and think better. I lost forty pounds and three dress sizes. But, best of all, I feel that I am better because of it all. I'm a lot different on the outside (I've actually got muscles!), but I'm different on the inside, too. More disciplined. More caring. A better caretaker of what God has given me.

A few months ago I discovered www.bodymedia.com, a company that produces a little monitor you wear on your arm. The gadget is like a pedometer on steroids, and it allows me to see how many calories I'm burning throughout my day and night. I'm still responsible for what I eat, but the body media device helps encourage me to move more and burn more calories. I love it.

So if the word *exercise* makes you cringe and think of sweat, pain, and smelly gym clothes, think of the word *fitness* instead. Fitness means being in shape to be your best. And being your best is beautiful.

Fitness Is Good, but More Is Not Better

Laura doesn't have to work out every day to keep her model's figure. There are several reasons why: First, she eats good foods that are part of a balanced diet; and second, she says living in New York is exercise enough. Working in New York City means lots of walking up and down city blocks, climbing stairs to the subway, and generally being caught up in the fast pace of life and being involved in a lot of sports.

Regardless of what you've heard about "going for the burn" and "no pain, no gain," exercise and fitness should not be excruciating. Exercise experts have realized that the "high impact" aerobics promoted years ago are actually harmful. One survey of twelve hundred aerobics students found that 43 percent had suffered damage to the back or knees and muscle aches and strains.

When you jump on one foot, for instance, the fragile bones and tendons in your foot are hit with a force equal to three times your body weight. That sends a shock wave up and down your body, and after a while, the body rebels.

Today experts recommend that aerobics not exceed thirty minutes, classes should not be taken more often than every other day, and no more than four hops should ever be performed in sequence on the same foot. Those who participate in aerobic dancing should also be careful to wear the proper shoes—running shoes are designed to take the impact on the heel and have heavy tread. Aerobic exercises, however, place most of the weight on the forward part of the foot, and shoes need a light tread so the foot is free to move in any direction.

Fitness Can Be Fun

Angie remembers being an absolute klutz in school. In the fifth grade her girls' phys ed class once broke into teams for a relay race. The object of the race was to dribble a basketball down an asphalt court, shoot a basket, and run back. Angie ran down and shot the ball thirty-two times before the team gave up and called her back.

Maybe P.E is a nightmare for you, too. Are you the last one chosen for team sports? Do you muddle through your phys. ed. classes and pray for the day when you don't have to take P.E. anymore? You can make athletics and fitness either a choice or a challenge — it all depends on your attitude. If you see sports and exercise as a way to improve yourself, activity will become fun. If you see it as just a lousy way to spend an hour, exercise will become a chore.

If you want to increase your fitness level, find an activity that you enjoy doing and make it a regular part of your day. And you don't have to suffer. All you really need to do is burn two hundred calories per day.

How do you burn two hundred calories? Choose two of the following activities. If you weigh 128 pounds (the more you weigh, the more calories you'll burn in a given time), you can burn one hundred calories by:

- Washing and waxing the car for 29 minutes
- Vigorously playing the piano for 26 minutes
- Polishing furniture for 52 minutes

- Vacuuming for 38 minutes
- Weeding the flower bed for 24 minutes
- Bowling for 34 minutes
- Dancing (fast!) for 10 minutes
- Playing Ping-Pong for 24 minutes
- Skating for 15 minutes
- Swimming for 20 minutes
- Playing volleyball for 34 minutes
- Jumping rope for 11 minutes
- Ironing for 52 minutes
- Standing for 48 minutes

See how easy it is to bring activity into your day? If you're in the marching band, the cross country team, or a cheerleader, you've already worked your fitness activity into your day. If you're not doing *something*, get out of that chair, turn off the television, and *move*. You'll be glad you did.

Fitness Is a Key to Weight loss

When it comes to weight loss and exercise, there are a few hard and fast formulas:

☐ If you exercise more and eat fewer calories, you'll lose weight.

☐ If you stay at the same exercise level and eat fewer calories, you'll lose weight.

☐ If you exercise more and eat the same calories as you're presently eating, you'll lose weight.

If you don't exercise and you lose weight, you're *very likely* to gain the weight back. Only 10 percent of all dieters who lose weight maintain their weight loss without increasing their exercise level.

How can exercise help you lose weight? First you should understand that a calorie is a unit of energy, and, as you know, food contains calories. Exercise is the only way to entice your body to "spend" the calories it has ingested, and you must burn off thirty-five hundred calories for every pound you want to lose.

Obviously, exercise burns calories. But regular exercise also decreases the appetite, and exercise "warms up" your body's engine so that it "runs" at a higher rate of speed for hours. So if you ride a stationary bike for half an hour in the morning, your body will burn more calories throughout the morning than if you hadn't exercised, even if you've done nothing but collapse into the TV chair.

People who exercise regularly have more energy than those who sit around all day. Exercise is mentally relaxing and helps you shed the everyday stress that enters your life. And though you may think you're too young to worry about health concerns, exercise can save your life. Dr. Thomas B. Gilliam, a professor of physical education at the University of Michigan, found that nearly half of four hundred high school students he studied had at least one factor for heart disease—high blood pressure, high cholesterol, or overweight — all of which could be reduced by increasing the students' physical activity.[1]

Walk Your Way to Fitness

What do Ralph Waldo Emerson, Henry David Thoreau, Thomas Jefferson, Abe Lincoln, and Harry Truman have in common? Aside from being great figures in US. history, all were walkers.

Maybe you didn't know that you burn about one hundred calories each mile you walk, *the same amount* of calories you'd burn jogging that mile. So unless you're in love with the feeling of running like the wind, try walking for fitness. Walking is a good aerobic exercise that requires your lungs to use oxygen more efficiently, plus it strengthens your heart and conditions your muscles. If you want to lose weight, walking can bum as much fat as jogging, and it's a safe, gradual exercise. Plus, walking is fun. You can walk with a friend or walk to have time to think by yourself. Walking requires no special equipment—only a good, comfortable pair of shoes. You can make the commitment to begin walking by promising to walk your dog a mile every other day. Both you and Fido will benefit!

If you're serious about walking, begin with a good stretch. Stretch your right calf gently by pressing your right heel to the ground and bending your left knee. Keep both knees pointing forward, then stretch the left calf in the same way. To stretch your quadriceps (the front muscle above your knees), with your left hand, pull your right foot behind you to your buttocks, keeping your right knee pointing straight to the ground. Hold for a minute, then repeat for the left quadriceps. Now you're ready to walk!

Begin by walking at a normal pace for five minutes, then for the next twenty to forty-five minutes walk briskly, swinging your arms easily. When you're ready to stop, slow down for the next five minutes to cool your body down and lower your pulse to its resting level. After your walk, repeat the stretches you performed earlier. Never bounce a tired muscle.

Schedule your walking program and gradually increase the time you spend walking. You might begin by walking three times a week, for thirty minutes a session. If you can't catch your breath, feel lightheaded or dizzy, or feel your heart pounding, slowdown!

Walking tips:

☐ Remember to drink at least eight to ten glasses of water each day to replace your body's water supply.

☐ If you walk at night, walk with a friend and wear reflectors and bright clothing so drivers can see you.

☐ If your neighborhood isn't safe or suitable for walking, walk a few laps around your shopping mall!

☐ Walk with your family. Walking time can be excellent mother/daughter or father/daughter bonding time.

☐ Always walk on smooth surfaces; you could trip or turn an ankle on a rough or unfamiliar pathway.

☐ Avoid neighborhoods or houses where barking dogs lurk — as every postal carrier knows, some dogs bite.

☐ Never walk in an unfamiliar place, and always tell someone at home where you are walking and what time you should return.

☐ Never walk with weights around your ankles — the added weight can injure your back. If you want to use weights, carry them in your hands or strapped around your wrists.

☐ If you're walking with a Walkman and you have music in your ears, be especially sensitive to traffic. Each year hundreds of walkers are hurt because they didn't hear the sound of a car's warning horn or the squeal of tires.

☐ Finally, for safe walking, always carry your some identification and change to make a phone call in an emergency.

Facts and Fiction

If you can't exercise every day, you shouldn't do it at all.

Not true. Regular exercise three times a week may be all you need.

Exercise will make me too tired.

Exercise actually gives you energy.

If an exercise doesn't hurt, it's not helping.

Exercise shouldn't hurt. You should push your limits, but not to the point of pain.

Wearing a plastic suit will help me sweat my weight off.

Dangerous. Plastic suits will not only dehydrate your body, but deprive your skin of needed oxygen. Wear natural cottons when exercising, and let your body cool naturally.

Instead of exercising thirty minutes, I figure ten minutes three times a day ought to do it.

Not true. Our bodies burn the readily accessible carbohydrates first, and don't begin to burn excess body fat until after about twenty minutes of exertion. So if you want to lose weight, you have to sustain the exercise for at least twenty minutes. But build up your endurance level slowly.

I can't walk in the winter, and I can't afford to join a gym so there's nothing I can do to stay fit.

Oh yes there is. You can find exercise programs on television that offer everything from body toning to aerobics. For very little money (save those babysitting funds!), you can purchase a stationary bike and pedal your way to fitness. Angie rides her stationary bike every morning while she reads her newspaper and watches the morning news on television. It's a great way to begin the day!

Sleeping Beauty

"Being a model requires looking good," says Laura, "and the way I look best is with plenty of sleep. All the makeup in the world can't change the way I feel, and I feel great when I'm rested."

Before we leave the subject of fitness, we think it's important that we stress not only *activity* but *inactivity* — namely, sleep. If you want to be your best, beautiful and healthy, you need to get enough sleep.

Sleep researcher Wilse Webb, from the University of Florida, says that if you wake up to an alarm clock every day, "you're shortening your natural sleep pattern."[2] In other words, your body is forced to wake up when it's not ready to awaken — and you could probably use more sleep.

Before the invention of the light bulb, the average person used to sleep about nine and a half hours every night. There was simply nothing else to do after sunset, so families went to bed early and rose with the sun. Today, however, prime time television lasts until eleven o'clock, there's homework to be done, phone calls to be made, plus round-the-clock-gotta-see movies on cable—when are we supposed to sleep?

Too many girls consider sleep expendable, something that's just not important. Besides, it's cool to wander into school, lean sleepily against a locker, and mumble, "I was up all night studying for my biology test. I only got three hours of sleep."

Bummer. Researchers have found that if you're sleep-deprived, your short-term memory will be impaired and you won't be as able to make good decisions or concentrate. Plus, while losing sleep one night will hurt you, losing sleep over several nights will nearly wreck you. Remember, it's during sleep that our bodies rest, our hair and nails grow, and our metabolism readjusts for another day.

How much sleep do you need? People vary in how much sleep they need, but most people require about seven to nine hours a night. If the alarm clock or your parents have to drag you from sleep every morning, try going to bed half an hour earlier. If you're still half-dead when it's time to get up the next morning, go to bed a full hour earlier.

Sometimes you can't help losing sleep, and on those days an afternoon nap of about an hour will really help. You really do need your beauty sleep!

If you have difficulty falling asleep on a regular basis, there are several things you can do to make yourself more ready for bed. First, get some exercise during the day so your body is ready for sleep. Second, don't drink coffee, colas, tea, or other soft drinks with caffeine after lunch. Just before bed, take a soothing warm bath or shower, drink a warm, caffeine-free tea with two teaspoons of honey, or eat a banana or other piece of fruit (the natural sugar will put you to sleep). Then settle down in bed with a boring or difficult book with the idea that if you don't fall asleep right away, everything's still all right. You'll probably be asleep before you know it. Whatever you do, don't--we repeat, *don't*--take a sleeping pill. They're dangerous, unhealthy and ultimately make a bad problem worse.

9

EATING FOR HEALTH AND BEAUTY

Wanda, another top model, has discovered that part of maintaining health and beauty is minding what we put—and don't put — into our bodies:

> Staying away from alcohol and cigarettes is my best beauty tip. They damage our bodies and age us prematurely. I also recommend plenty of sleep. It works wonders!

Food, glorious food. Don't care what it looks like!" sang the orphans in the hit musical *Oliver.* Today we Americans aren't starving, and we *do* care what our food looks like; we just don't care what food is doing to our bodies.

But with the emphasis on eating "lite" and good nutrition, maybe we're learning to care. We should be learning. In our country today we have more foods available than anywhere on the earth. You could drive right now to your grocery story and buy practically anything you want. We have "real" foods and "fake" foods, with artificial sugars, fats, and tastes. At a fast food drive-in you can buy a burger laden with calories or a low-fat version made from seaweed or soybeans.

Dr. Charles Kuntzleman has estimated that the average U.S. citizen has more than three thousand calories cross his or her plate every day. That's fifteen hundred to two thousand pounds of food per year — specifically: 16 pounds of boxed cereal
280 eggs
175 pounds of fruit 70 pounds of bread
250 pounds of vegetables 230 pounds of meat and fish
430 gallons of soft drinks 144 gallons of milk and cream 560 cups of coffee
150 cups of tea 130 pounds of fat 100 pounds of sugar 9 pounds of salt![1]

And guess what? Despite the tremendous amount of food available to us, we are not eating well.

What Should We Eat?

Our bodies are wonders of creation, incredibly designed in intricate ways that scientists and nutritionists are still exploring. The best analogy we can use to describe our bodies is to compare them to a car—you may be a luxury model, a compact, or something in between, but you've still got an engine and your motor still requires the proper fuel!

Foods are the fuel our bodies need to function. If you fill a high-performance car with a watered-down version of gasoline, you're going to have a car that sputters and stops along the way. Likewise, if you fill your metabolic engine with junk foods that don't meet your nutritional requirements, prepare for sputtering and stopping. In other words, you're likely to run out of energy or even get sick.

The Food Pyramid and "MyPlate"

The U.S. Agriculture Department once issued a new guide to eating and called it the "Food Pyramid." Basically, the pyramid broke foods down into five groups (instead of the old "basic four" food groups) and recommended a certain number of daily servings from each group.

Of the foundational group, the bread group, you should eat six to eleven servings per day. A serving might be one slice of bread, one ounce of cereal, or one-half cup of rice or pasta. As you select your bread choices, remember that whole-wheat products have more fiber, minerals, and vitamins than the highly refined flour found in white bread. Also keep in mind that croissants, granola, and waffles are usually higher in fat and calories than other bread choices. And while Twinkies, cookies, pies, and doughnuts are made of flour, they are so high in fats, sugar, and calories that they are not good bread choices.

Fruits and vegetables made up the second level of the food pyramid, and experts recommended that we eat three to five servings of vegetables and two to four servings of fruit every day. A serving was one-half cup of chopped vegetables or one cup of raw leafy vegetables such as lettuce. One medium apple, banana, or orange, one-half cup of chopped fruit, or three-fourths of a cup of fruit juice counted as one serving of fruit.

Fruits and vegetables are rich in vitamins and minerals. Whenever possible, eat fruits and vegetables raw, fresh from the produce department. Fruits and vegetables that have been canned usually have too much salt added, and the high temperatures necessary for canning destroy many valuable vitamins. If fresh fruits and vegetables are not available, try frozen foods before resorting to canned.

The third level of the food pyramid contained the milk group (two to three daily servings needed) and the protein group (two to three daily servings needed). Even though your parents may not ask you to drink milk every day, you still need it. If you've never been wild about the taste of white milk, you can still get your important calcium and B vitamins in cheese, yogurt, ice milk, and other dairy products. Just remember to make wise choices. Instead of the calorie-laden and fat-heavy ice cream dessert, opt for frozen yogurt. Your body will thank you!

The protein group in the food pyramid included beef, fish, pork, and poultry. As you make selections from this group, remember that beef and pork are higher in fat and calories than poultry, and protein foods that are fried are much higher in calories and fat than those that are broiled, baked, or boiled.

The final level, the tiny top of the pyramid, contained the oils, sweets, and fats. These were not a bona fide food group, and should be used sparingly. Your body needs a daily dose of oil/fat, but you're probably getting plenty without having to add any. Look at the wrapper of the next candy bar you eat, and you'll be surprised to see how many fat grams you've just eaten. Fats don't just hide in candy, either. A Burger King Whopper contains thirty-eight fat grams, and a McDonald's Big Mac offers forty-four. One-fourth of a medium Domino's Cheese Pizza, on the other hand, has only six fat grams.

In 2011, however, the government left the food pyramid behind in favor of "MyPlate," which split a round plate into four sections: one part fruit, one part vegetable, one part protein, one part grains. A small circle, representing dairy, sat off to the side, exactly where you might place a glass of milk. I'm sure government officials were thinking that it's easier to eat healthy meal-by-meal than to try and plan an entire day's eating at once. I've a hunch they were right.

For more information, visit http://choosemyplate.com.

Whether you use "MyPlate" or the food pyramid, do try to eat from all the different food groups each day.

Drinking for Beauty

You may not realize it, but what you drink contributes as much to your diet as what you eat. Most teenagers and adults drink soft drinks by the gallon, while fruit juices and coffee are also popular beverages. But the most important liquid you can drink is water.

When Laura moved to Paris to begin her modeling career, she noticed that her desire for sodas decreased. Coke and other sodas weren't as common in France as they are in the United States, and restaurants serve them with very little ice, so they aren't cold. "It was easy to break the habit of four sodas a day," Laura says. After returning from Paris, Laura went three years without a soda and never felt better. "I learned to drink natural fruit juices and water," she says. "Once you get in the habit of drinking good things, sodas don't taste good anymore. They're too sweet."

Nearly 70 percent of your body is water. Next to air, water is the most important thing you need to survive. You could live for several weeks without food, but you could survive only a few days without water.

How much water have you drunk today? If you're like most people, you haven't drunk nearly enough. Sure, you do get some water in your foods, colas, and fruit juices, but your body would *love* a glass of pure, sparkling water right about now. You should be drinking between eight and ten glasses of pure water every day. Dr. Leroy Perry has developed a formula to figure the minimum amount of water you need, based on your body weight. The active teenager should figure one-half her body weight to equal the ounces of water needed daily. For instance, if you weigh one hundred twenty pounds, you need half of one hundred twenty—that's sixty ounces of water, or about seven eight-ounce glasses of water every day.[2]

Water is necessary for those basic bodily functions you never think about. When your kidneys remove wastes from your cells, those wastes must be dissolved in water. If there isn't enough water in your body, your kidneys may be damaged. Water also carries nutrients and oxygen to the cells, it helps keep your body cool through perspiration, and water lubricates your joints and mucous membranes.

Water is also essential for beauty. A healthy supply of water keeps hair supple, skin smooth, and eyes sparkling and bright. Many women who spend a fortune on creams and lotions to keep their skin smooth could accomplish the same effect just by drinking water to moisturize their skin from the *inside*.

Our bodies are constantly losing water through perspiration, urination, and even through breathing. You lose about a pint of water every day just by exhaling. In hot weather, or when you're exercising or working hard, the amount of water your body loses increases incredibly. If you don't drink enough water, you're hampering your body's efforts from the beginning. You're like a race car driver who fills his car's gas tank but forgets to make sure the engine has oil. Sometime during the race, that car engine is going to overheat and burn up.

Drinking lots of water helps your body burn fats, so if you're trying to lose weight, you should drink lots of water. "Proper water intake is the key to weight loss," says Dr. Donald Robertson, director of the Southwest Bariatrics Nutrition Center in Scottsdale, Arizona. "If people who are trying to lose weight don't drink enough water, the body can't metabolize the fat, they retain fluid, which keeps the weight up, and the whole procedure that we're trying to set up falls apart."[3]

Did you catch an important truth? If you don't drink enough water, your body will actually *retain* water, a problem for many girls during the week of and before their menstrual cycle. So, if you tend to gain weight around "that time of the month," you'll be able to stave off a lot of menstrual bloating if you simply drink more water and avoid salty foods (salt encourages the body to retain water).

Why can't you just drink ten or twelve Diet Cokes and count

them as water? Because, while other beverages do contain water, they also contain substances that are not healthy. For instance, caffeinated beverages stimulate the adrenal glands, while fruit juices contain a lot of sugar and stimulate the pancreas. Soda contains sodium. So these drinks don't *help* the body, they *work* the body, because your stomach and glands have to go to work digesting the other substances contained in those drinks.[4] Plus, if you fill up on juices and colas, you won't have the thirst or desire to drink more water.

What kind of water should you drink? Any kind will do, but watch out for sparkling waters that have other "added" ingredients. If water from your kitchen sink doesn't taste good, ask your folks about installing an inexpensive and easy-to-use water filter. And nothing tastes better than ice-cold water, so keep a huge jug in the refrigerator and develop the habit of reaching for it as readily as you reach for those two-liter bottles of Pepsi.

Balancing the Body Beautiful

We almost hate to talk about *dieting* because frankly, we can't see what you look like. We don't know what you should weigh, but we do know that most girls think they're too heavy when they're just right. We can give you guidelines, and we hope you'll go by them, but we want to stress *that your ideal body size and shape may not be model-thin.* Your ideal body may not be like your best friend's. But it is still right for you.

Standards of beauty have changed over the years from the curvaceous Marilyn Monroe standard to the unisex slim Jane Fonda type. For instance, Miss Sweden of 1951 was five feet seven inches tall and weighed 151 pounds; the 1983 Miss Sweden was five feet nine inches tall and weighed 109 pounds.[5]

How much should you weigh? There are several "formulas" currently in vogue, but Dr. Reuben Andres recently published a revised table of healthy weight ranges for women. No one can be dogmatic about this topic for you, but grab a calculator and give this formula a try:

1.   Divide your height, in inches, by 66. (For instance, five feet nine inches equals 69 inches, divided by 66 equals 1.045.)

2.   Multiply the result by itself.

3.   Multiply that result by your age plus 100.

4.   That number is the *middle* of your healthy weight range.

If you are within fifteen pounds of this number, either higher or lower, your weight is fine.[6]

Where do you fall in your ideal weight range? If you are more than fifteen pounds over that middle weight, or more than fifteen pounds under, you should know that being *overweight* is just as unhealthy as being *underweight*. And no matter what you weigh, you should consult the food pyramid and begin to eat a well-balanced diet. If you need to gain weight, add more daily servings, particularly from the lower groups such as bread, fruits, and vegetables. If you need to lose weight, cut your calories back, but never go below twelve hundred calories per day. You need at least that many to keep your body's engine running smoothly.

Successful Weight Loss

Before you begin a "diet," ask yourself if you are really overweight. By whose standards are you judging yourself? If you are dieting only so you'll wear a smaller size or so you'll look like your sister or your best friend, or if you're dieting just to look good for one special occasion, you're dieting for the wrong reasons. Maybe you shouldn't be "dieting" at all. Remember, if your weight falls within fifteen pounds of the middle weight you determined from our formula, your weight is *fine*.

However, if you really need to lose weight, don't think of yourself as on a "diet." If you consider your new way of eating a diet, it will be something to "go on" and "come off" as the mood strikes. Take it from us, that's no way to live. If you want to lose weight, you must make permanent changes in your eating patterns.

Like Laura, Angie was a tall and skinny string bean throughout her high school and college years. She was active and ate like a horse, but weight never clung to her. But once she began to work at home, with the refrigerator and pantry close at hand, the excess pounds crept on.

First she tried a medically supervised diet program that limited her to seven hundred calories a day. It was an expensive program that required weighing in at a medical clinic three times a week, but she lost twenty pounds. In two years, though, those twenty pounds came back and increased to thirty.

Angie then tried drinking powdered diet formulas at home, but after a breakfast and lunch of the murky stuff, she was ravenous. The "sensible dinner" she was supposed to eat turned into a free-for-all. "I'll be good tomorrow" was her favorite saying.

After her weight ballooned to the point where she could no longer wear even her "fat" clothes, Angie tried the all-American weight loss program, Weight Watchers®. We're not intending to give a commercial plug here, but Weight Watchers® offers a well-rounded nutritional program that you can follow/or *life*. The program includes an emphasis on exercise, group support, and the variety of being able to eat restaurant foods, home foods, or prepackaged foods.

"It was a great program because if I wanted a piece of chocolate cake, I could have my piece of chocolate cake," Angie says. "I just couldn't have the *whole* cake. I realized I was going to have to make eating changes for the rest of my life, and Weight Watchers® taught me how to make those changes."

If you are interested in losing weight, whether it's ten pounds or one hundred, we suggest you call your local Weight Watchers® chapter and inquire about their meetings. Weekly meetings give you group support and suggestions, the weekly fee will keep you serious and dedicated to your goal (why is it we always appreciate things more if we pay for them?), and the program is healthy and versatile.

If you decide to modify your eating habits on your own, don't think you can lose your weight quickly or easily with the help of pills. Diet pills contain phenylpropanolamine (PPA), a drug that works like the amphetamine speed. These pills may temporarily curb your appetite, but they can also cause high blood pressure, kidney damage, hallucinations, and even *fatal* strokes.[7]

The best weight-reduction programs are those that take weight off *slowly*, through a combination of good eating and exercise. The slower you take the excess weight off, the more likely you are to keep it off, in part because you'll form good nutritional habits. Anyone can starve herself to lose a few pounds, but we all have to eat, and unless you change your harmful eating patterns, you'll only regain the weight you lose and more.

"Bummer!" you may be thinking. "Can dieting really make me fat?" The answer is a resounding *yes*. Earlier we compared your body to a car, and that analogy works well here, too. You see, like a car's engine, our bodies all "idle" at different speeds. Some of us are slow and calm, and we have a slow metabolism that burns calories slowly. Other people are hyper—you've seen them. They jiggle their feet even when they're sitting still. These people have "fast" metabolic engines, and they burn calories like a hot oven.

But your body is a lot smarter than a car. If you begin to withhold food from your body, your "engine" begins to idle at a reduced speed. "Wait a minute here, we're in the middle of a famine!" your body thinks, so it burns less calories even when you're resting. And when you do eat, your body hoards calories, storing up because it senses that famine may return any time. The more often you "feast and starve," the better your body be comes at burning calories slowly and storing the food you do give it.

Dieting slows your metabolism and your body learns to function with less food. The more severe your food deprivation, the more your body slows down. That's why extremely low calorie diets are dangerous. You may feel tired, grumpy, and if you eat even one little thing that's a "forbidden" food, you'll gain weight amazingly fast.

Angie found that she lost weight faster and with less "suffering" when she ate at least twelve hundred calories a day than when she ate only seven hundred calories a day. Plus, your body burns a lot of calories simply by digesting food, and one of the best ways to rev the metabolic engine is to eat. Just be sure you're eating good foods like raw fruits, lean meats, and vegetables — not Twinkies!

Geoffrey Cannon and Hetty Einzig explain it this way:

> What the diet books don't stress is this important concept: Dieting slows the body's metabolism, while regular physical exercise speeds it up. Thus, for the sedentary person, a lifetime spent on and between diets will be self-defeating. Habitual dieters are on a downward spiral that remorselessly defeats their efforts. Indeed, studies indicate that each new diet may train the body to become more energy efficient, require less food, and use less oxygen.
>
> We become fit and healthy not simply by deprivation but by using all our energies. As additional muscle tissue is built up with exercise, we develop a faster metabolic rate. The body gradually adapts by losing fat and gaining lean tissue, allowing us to eat our fill without gaining weight.[8]

Facts and Fiction

Bread and potatoes are fattening.

Not true. One slice of regular bread contains eighty calories; the average baked potato has only 105. It's what we put *on* the bread and potato that are fattening, so learn to eat them with reduced calorie margarine, with fruit only spreads, or plain.

All calories are created equal, so it really doesn't matter where my calories come from.

Not true. One ounce of fat contains 255 calories, while one ounce of protein contains 113 calories. So the tiny bit of butter is calorie-dense, and you'd have to eat bowls and bowls of salad to equal the calories in one tiny ounce of butter. Plus, the body doesn't have to work to store the fat calories — they're ready to go right on your hips or wherever. Fat is fat. But the calories in a carrot, for instance, have to be converted by your body engine in order to be stored, and your body will burn energy just trying to do that.

Fruits are low-calorie, so I can eat as many as I want.

Sometimes. Some fruits are low-calorie, but some aren't. And while it will always be better and more filling if you munch on an apple instead of a Three Musketeers Bar, still, it is possible to overindulge on fruits.

The quicker you lose weight, the better off you'll be.

Not true. The quicker the weight comes off, the sooner it will come back on. Plus, low-calorie diets deplete your body's muscle mass instead of burning fat, and it's dangerous for your body to swing back and forth between weight extremes. Exercise, which builds muscle mass, and slow weight reduction are the way to go.

Just this one little bite won't hurt me . . .

Maybe it won't. But your body doesn't forget what you put in it. Angie used to tell herself that eating raw cookie dough didn't count in her daily calories, because the cookies weren't officially baked. Some women think they can overlook nibbles, bites from other people's plates, and leftovers. But your body keeps merciless track of what you store inside.

Just by cutting out one can of sugared cola a day, you could lose fifteen pounds in a year. By eating one extra piece of chocolate cake a *week,* you would gain five pounds in a year. By cutting out one small cake doughnut every day, you would lose twenty-four pounds in a year. Pretty amazing, isn't it? Little things do count.

Learn to take shortcuts and save on calories you won't even miss. Order your Burger King Whopper without mayonnaise and you'll save one hundred fifty-nine calories (season burgers with mustard instead). Order a McDonald's Big Mac without the sauce, and you'll save 105 calories. Indulge in a Pizza Hut pizza without meat (try loading it with mushrooms, green peppers, and onions!), and you'll save up to 144 calories, plus you'll be adding valuable veggies to your diet. If you go to a salad bar and squirt your creation with the juice of a lemon instead of ladling on the dressing, you'll save up to 133 calories.

Better yet, avoid McDonald's, Burger King, and Pizza Hut altogether and the weight will come off more easily. Unless you have the dedication to eat only the fast-food garden salads, why subject yourself to temptation?

Weight Obsession

As recently as the 1930s, some women used a pill that introduced a tapeworm into their system.[9] Why? Because tapeworms eat the food in your digestive system. These women saw it as a way to stay thin.

If that sounds gross and repulsive, it's really no worse or more dangerous than some of the things girls do today to remain slender. Too many girls are so obsessed with food and their weight that they develop anorexia nervosa or bulimia. The trouble is that we don't really see ourselves as others do, and you can be thin and still think of yourself as a fat person.

Anorexia is a serious ailment that most often affects young girls who literally starve themselves to death. The singer Karen Carpenter, whose voice was like velvet, died young because her body never recovered from the way she starved it.

Many people feel that anorexia is a disease that originates in the mind, but other researchers have found that anorexics have a common deficiency in zinc. Zinc, a mineral, helps the body maintain an appetite and helps us to taste and smell foods. While no one knows if the zinc deficiency is a cause or result of anorexia, zinc supplements have helped many girls regain their appetites.[10]

Bulimia is similar to anorexia because those who suffer from it are preoccupied with fears of being fat, but bulimics are more likely to binge on foods, then "purge," or simply throw up the food they have eaten. Some girls act like purging is the greatest diet idea to ever come along, but purging can kill you. Your body, throat, and stomach were not meant to throw up on demand, and bulimia can lead to serious health problems.

The acid in your stomach is strong enough to digest food, so it's also strong enough to eat your skin and tear the enamel off your teeth. Excessive vomiting forces this strong stomach acid into your esophagus, which causes pain and swelling in the throat. After a period of time one runs the risk of not only tearing the throat, but rupturing the esophagus. Also, the more you vomit, the more scar tissue is built up in the esophagus, causing your throat to narrow. This makes it extremely difficult and painful to swallow.[11]

If you or someone you know suffers from anorexia or bulimia, please tell a trusted adult or your parents today. You may also consider calling one of the following organizations for information and help. You deserve to be happy with yourself, so give these numbers a call *today:*

ANAD: The National Association of Anorexia Nervosa and Associated Disorders (708) 831-3438.

American Anorexia/Bulimia Association, Inc. (212) 734-1114.

The Ten Commandments of Nutrition for Balanced Beauty

1. *Thou shalt never,* ever take diet pills, water pills, laxatives, or go on fad diets.

2. *Thou shalt never* skip breakfast. (The best way to get your body's internal engine humming after a nighttime fast of nine or ten hours is to eat a generous breakfast. It's the absolute *best* way to start your day.)

3. *Thou shalt carry* a healthy snack to munch on when you are hungry. *(Healthy* snack, we said. If you feed your stomach when it rumbles, you'll keep your internal engine chugging happily along, plus you won't be as likely to overindulge at the next meal. Try healthy snacks like raw veggies, peanuts, granola, raisins, dried fruits, or unsalted nuts.)

4. *Thou shalt eat* lots of foods with fiber. (Fiber is found in wheat breads, fruits, and vegetables. It's the skin on a baked potato, the green fibers in lettuce. Fiber is literally tough stuff, so it fills up your tummy and keeps you from being hungry twenty minutes after you rise from the table.)

5.   ***Thou shalt eat*** foods cooked the "B" for beauty way: baked, broiled, or boiled (not fried). In other words, avoid fast food.

6.   *Thou shalt obey* thy doctor and eat your fruits and veggies.

7.   *Thou shalt drink at least* eight glasses of water a day.

8.   *Thou shalt limit* sweet treats to two or three a week. (Life would be no fun without at least a little chocolate!)

9.   *Thou shalt never* add salt to anything. Our foods are salty enough!

10.   *Thou shalt remember* that nutrition is to be tackled one day at a time. If you goof up today, you can do better tomorrow. But don't make this a reason to celebrate a "last supper" every night.

10
BEAUTY IS AN ATTITUDE

We've nearly reached the end of our book, and we've given you tips on your hair, your toes, and nearly everything in between. But did you know that you may have the face of a goddess and do everything we suggest and still be only halfway beautiful? For beauty is more than how you look, how you walk, or what you eat. Beauty is an attitude.

Beauty probably isn't the attitude you expect it to be. Beauty isn't snobby: "Look at me, I'm the most gorgeous girl in the room." Beauty is instead a quiet attitude that says, "I'm confident because I accept the way God made me. Confident enough to laugh and be free and sure of who I am."

Beauty's attitude doesn't worry if other girls are pretty. Beauty's attitude isn't jealous or competitive. Beauty's attitude is born of knowing who, what, and why you are.

Krista Marcy, another model friend of Laura's, says, "When you're a model, you often hear, 'Oh, you're so beautiful.' But there are so many beautiful girls out there. When I'm working, I try to radiate the beauty that comes from knowing God. When someone tells me I'm beautiful, I know they've seen so many pretty girls that what's caught their eye is the difference on the inside--the inner beauty God has given me."

What Beauty Is
How would you define physical beauty? Years ago, curvaceous women who carried more than a few "extra" pounds by today's

standards were considered beautiful. In medieval history, the standard of beauty required blonde hair and blue eyes, and brunettes were thought less than beautiful. Cindy Crawford might have had a hard time in the Middle Ages!

Fortunately, the beauty standard of today allows for a wide variety in hair, eye, and skin colors. Linda Evangelista, a top model, has changed her hair color several times, and she's been in demand as everything from a redhead to a blonde to a brunette. The color of your hair, skin, or eyes doesn't matter as much as you may think. Beauty is within your reach.

> I found my most impressive beauty tip in the Bible. In Deuteronomy 28,1 read that if I obey the Lord, the One who originated all beauty, He would command blessings on all I set my hands to do. So as I set my hands to my hair, my skin, or even my nails, I stand on this promise, believing that God will prosper even these simple things.
> -Wanakee

Some goofy comic once said, "Beauty is skin deep, but ugliness goes down to the bone." While beauty may be hard to define, ugly isn't. What's ugly? Severe acne, extreme obesity, stringy hair, listless skin, slumping posture. In other words, *unhealthy* is unattractive. *A lack of proper self-esteem* is unappealing. The good news is that you can beat both. You can get help for medical and weight problems, and you can develop confidence in yourself.

"There's a big gap between gorgeous and ugly," says J. Kevin Thompson, an associate professor of psychology at the University of South Florida. "Most of us fall in that middle range of acceptability. People won't walk away from us because of our looks, and we won't be turned down for jobs. Instead of looking great, we look good, but good is passable."[1]

Hey, looking good is great. We may not all be models, but we can look good and we can be our best. Don't let yourself fall victim to the ads or commercials that promise if you'll just drink the right diet cola or wear the right perfume, guys will be falling over themselves to hand you a towel at the beach. It just isn't going to happen. We don't all have model's bodies.

Many girls fall into a trap of believing that beauty is only an external quality measured by how they compare to the supermodels they see in fashion magazines or on TV. From many years of experience, Laura knows that even though one may have the sought-after outside packaging, without elements of inner beauty one can be very unattractive. Some models she has worked with, though gorgeous on the outside, are constantly insecure, self-centered, unstable, confused, and even lonely.

Maybe you've watched the Olympics on television or seen a concert pianist perform. We all love to admire the tremendous skill and discipline of these talented people, but we don't all assume that with just a little work we can perform like they can. We know they arrived at their present level of expertise after years of work and practice. They have special abilities that we may never be able to match.

Just like those performers, the models you see on television and in ads have special bodies. Models are 9 percent taller and 16 percent thinner than the average person. Research by Jennifer Brenner at Boston University found that American models are an average five feet, nine-and-a-half inches tall and weigh about 122.8 pounds. The average American woman at five feet, four inches is five inches shorter and several pounds heavier.[2]

In fact, advertising people will audition *hundreds* of girls to find one they can "pass off" as perfect. Those commercial ad images you gasp at and envy are the result of thousands of dollars and many hours of labor. Laura says that after being on even one of these sets, you realize how artificial, "unreal," and almost unbelievable the final product really is. Beauty lighting, professional makeup and hair-styling, camera angles, filters, retouching, and every other trick in the book are used to create that attractive image you see. No one looks like that without a lot of help, money, and Photoshop, and no one looks like that every day.

Laura, who has enjoyed a career as a top fashion model, is five feet, nine inches tall and weighs 123 pounds. Angie, whose job is writing books, is five feet, nine inches tall and 140 pounds. Laura has small bones; she has the ideal body for professional modeling. While Angie is tall, she does not have, nor ever will have, the body or skills to be a model. She weighs a comfortable and healthy weight for her height and is happy doing what she does best.

We want you to understand this: You don't have to look like a cover girl to be beautiful; you only have to be the best you can be.

You need only concentrate on enhancing the gifts God has given you. Don't worry about trying to look like someone else.

We know that some girls will do anything to become models. Laura cautions girls and their parents to beware of wasting money in pursuit of the modeling dream. Thousands of schools, scams, and photographers wait to take money from star-struck wannabes. She suggests getting professional advice before spending any money on schooling, photos, or composites.

If you're considering a modeling career, seek the advice of working professionals first. CONTACT is an organization of such people. They provide honest, comprehensive, and current information about the modeling business. To reach them, write or call: CONTACT, P.O. Box 172, New York, NY, 10044; 212935-8489.

You Don't Have to Be a Slave to Beauty

How much time did you spend last week on your personal beauty? Be honest. Add up the minutes you spent in the shower, standing in front of your closet to find something to wear, time doing (or undoing) your nails, the minutes you stood waving the blow dryer or fussing with hair curlers, the time you spent exercising (or making excuses for not exercising), the hours you spent at the mall shopping for the perfect accessory, the time you spent reading the latest fashion magazines (and this book!), shaving your legs, tweezing your brows, and brushing your teeth.

Maybe you spent only the minimum of time on your own personal beauty. Or maybe you spent hours and hours making yourself look better.

We wrote this book to help you make the most of the time you spend to be your best. We don't want you to waste your time, for time is the stuff life is made of, and you don't want to waste your life worrying about whether or not your eye makeup is on straight!

That may sound silly, but a lot of women have a lopsided view of what beauty is and what it should be. We are preoccupied with our bodies, and too often we think we will never be happy unless we are *perfect*. Not one of us is or ever will be perfect. Even the models you see on television and in ads aren't perfect. Many of those super-skinny models have had to resort to dangerous, un-healthy breast implants to get womanly curves on those thin bod-ies, and that skinny, busty look isn't healthy or fit — it's totally artificial. Other models have what it takes because they're born with a certain body type and they work hard to keep it.

> I used to scan the magazines and look at pictures of beautiful people. I'd take their best physical characteristics and mix those with the personalities of charming people I met I tried to be like them and couldn't. I felt ugly in comparison, inside and out. One day I met the Lord Jesus Christ and asked Him to be my personal Lord and Savior, and then I saw His beauty shine within my heart. He changed my whole attitude about myself in a beautiful way.
> -Claudia McClintock

Will Beauty Bring Happiness?

We're surrounded by images of smiling, beautiful people on television, in movies, and in magazines, and it would be easy to get the idea that all beautiful people are successful, happy, rich, and in love.

But all the so-called "beautiful" people aren't successful, rich, in love, or happy. And not all people who are happy and in love are cover-girl beautiful. Believe it or not, the Bible talks a lot about beauty; in fact, the words *beauty, beautiful,* and *well-favored* occur seventy-eight times in the God's Word. The Bible tells us that Israel's high priests wore garments made for "glory and for beauty" (Ex. 28:2 God commanded them to *look good!*), Absalom was one of the most beautiful men who ever lived (but his beauty literally went to his head), Esther became queen because she was stunningly beautiful (and as queen she saved her entire nation), and beauty is found in the Lord and His holiness.

So from the Scriptures we learn that beauty can be used for good or bad. Some of the strongest people in the Bible (David and Esther, for instance) were beautiful, and so were some of the worst (the prostitutes of Jerusalem).

But you don't have to be drop-dead gorgeous for God to use you. Think for a moment about Jesus, God's Son. He was the Creator of the universe in human form. All power was given to Him. Was He beautiful, or handsome, as we think of beauty?

Surely He had loving eyes, strong hands, and lips that spoke of

113

love and compassion. He was probably lean and tanned from spending time in the sun, and we know He wore a beard. He probably had brown hair and deep brown eyes. We know people flocked to Him, children loved Him, men admired Him, women cherished Him, the sick trusted Hm.

Was He beautiful? To us who have never seen Him, Jesus is the most beautiful, loving man who ever walked the earth. We say that because we know the beauty that exists *within* Jesus Christ. But the Bible tells us that Jesus "had no beauty or majesty to attract us to him, nothing in his appearance that we should desire him" (Isa. 53:2).

Physically, Jesus was not a poster hunk. He did not stand head and shoulders above the crowd. If He were walking the earth today, He wouldn't be featured in **GQ**. As far as physical beauty goes, Jesus was an ordinary man.

But how He outshone other men. The love and concern from His eyes drew people to Him. He walked with the confidence of a man who knows why He lives and who controls His life. Jesus may not have been beautiful on the outside; He was beautiful from the inside out. People saw the difference, and their lives were changed by it.

> Inner beauty is what lights up a room and what attracts others to you. My relationship with Christ and knowing I'm forgiven is the main ingredient in my inner beauty. Inner beauty is long lasting and improves with age, unlike outer beauty that fades. I love what Proverbs 31:30 says. "Charm is deceptive, and beauty is fleeting; but a woman who fears the Lord is to be praised."
> -Ali Winslow

The Bible tells us that we should concentrate on inner beauty. In 1 Peter 3:3-4, we read:

> Your beauty should not come from outward adornment, such as braided hair and the wearing of gold jewelry and fine clothes. Instead, it should be that of your inner self, the unfading beauty of a gentle and quiet spirit, which is of great worth in

God's sight.

Some people have interpreted this verse to mean that women should never wear jewelry or makeup or elaborate hairstyles. But if you follow that logic, women should never wear fine clothes, either, and there certainly are times when it is appropriate to put on our best. The virtuous woman described in Proverbs 31 had beautiful clothes, and she wore them to enhance her grace and beauty.

Peter was telling women that we shouldn't concentrate on *what we wear* as much as we focus on *who we are on the inside.* Outer beauty is fine and certainly has its place, but inner beauty is so much more important.

You can be beautiful from the inside out. No matter what your outside is like, you can turn your life over to the God who designed you and decide right now to be what God wants you to be. True beauty begins there.

> I've seen some beautiful people become very ugly and some seemingly unattractive people be truly beautiful. When we allow God's perfect love to be reflected in our lives, we become more beautiful than we could ever hope to be on our own. This beauty is everlasting!
> -Megan

Finding Inner Beauty

In Taiwan, girls who wished to compete for the Miss China 1992 crown were asked to comfort the dying, give backrubs to homeless people, and play with orphans. According to pageant officials, the "inner beauty" campaign was launched to counter criticism that beauty pageant contestants were vain and arrogant. A spokesman for the organization said that contestants must prove they have virtues other than mere good looks. Beauty, the Chinese have recognized, should be found on the inside as well as the outside.[3]

How can you find your own inner beauty? First of all, put yourself in touch with the God who created you. If there has been a time in your life when you accepted Jesus Christ as your Lord and Savior, it shouldn't be hard to pray and ask His guidance in this area of beauty.

But if you have never been introduced to Jesus as a **personal** Savior, we need to talk a moment about who He is. Did you know that God, the ruler and Creator of the universe, loves you more than any person on earth ever could? Because He loves you so much, He wants to be your friend. A real, living, loyal friend.

But we humans have a problem. We're not like God. We're not morally perfect. We're prone to failure and rebellion and doing things that aren't at all godly. That's called sin, and sin creates a huge gap between us and the God who loves us. We could never, ever hope to become good enough to cross over that gap on our own. Going to church won't make you good enough, praying all day won't do it, even giving all your money to worthy causes doesn't add up to holiness from God's viewpoint.

Without Christ, the Bible states the penalty for our sins is "death" (Rom. 6:23), which is eternal separation from God; the Bible calls it "hell." The Bible clearly points to Christ as the only bridge over the gap that sin creates between us and God.

Sounds pretty hopeless, doesn't it? It's not. God knew we could never be perfect, so He sent His Son, Jesus, who was born from a virgin mother and who actually lived a perfect, sinless life on earth. He went through everything we go through—loneliness, hurt, pain, temptation, betrayal but He never gave in to bitterness. He never told a lie. He never rebelled against God's plan. He never sinned.

Jesus was put to death on a cruel cross, even though He had done nothing to deserve it. While He hung on the cross, He took the penalty for our sins, and though He didn't deserve to die, He did. He died so that you and I could have eternal life. He defeated death when He came back to life three days later.

When we accept Jesus and His sacrifice, God forgives us for our sin and can then become our Savior, and there is no longer a gap between us and God. Then we become His children and He our Lord and best friend, and He guarantees us a home in heaven.

When we decided we wanted to be God's children, we talked to Him that's prayer and told Him something like this:

> Lord Jesus, I realize that I have done things that are wrong, and I need Your forgiveness. I want You to be my Savior, and I invite You into my life, to change me and make me the kind of

person You want me to be. Thank You for helping me!

But simply reciting the prayer isn't what makes you one of God's children. We accept Jesus as our Lord and Savior through *faith* — we *choose* to accept Him and give Him control of our lives. It's a conscious decision you make, and no one else can make it for you.

Without Christ's forgiveness, our sin makes us ugly on the inside. All the "cover-up" remedies in the world can't change that. God sees it and others will eventually see it. Only Christ can make us beautiful in God's sight. True inner beauty begins with God at the center of our lives and grows outward.

Being a child of God is great. We asked Jesus to be our Savior years ago, and we've found that He's a real friend. He understands when you feel guilty, sad, or hurt. He helps us handle the hard times and gives us wisdom when things aren't going right. And He is the One who makes us beautiful on the inside, because He brings love, joy, peace, and hope to our lives. And when your smile and your eyes fill up with those truly valuable qualities, you can't help but shine.

> Inner beauty is a quality that comes from knowing God personally. It shines from the heart, and only He can light it up.
> -Sara Richmond

Beauty Begins in Quiet Confidence

When your beauty is rooted on the inside, your outside will begin to change. Kaylan Pickford was a housewife who didn't even wear makeup until she was forty-three years old. At forty-five, she began modeling, and six years later she was a top model in New York City. In her book, *Always Beautiful,* she writes:

> A woman who feels beautiful and loved can radiate Beauty. . . You have to know who and what you are and claim beauty for yourself. Even when you are in fantastic physical shape and groom yourself beautifully, you can't just sit around and wait for outside approval.

People did not seek me out as a beauty until I started treating myself differently—positively—in my uniqueness, until I made the decision to find and accept myself at my best without comparing myself to the beauty of youth or the beauty of others. Comparisons can be deadly and damaging. Don't do that to yourself. While choosing to see the beauty in anyone or anything can't possibly diminish your life, it also includes discovering your own particular beauty. You are an original — miraculously unique.[4]

"I'll never be beautiful!" you may be saying to yourself. "I'm an original, all right. An original ugly."

Don't feel alone. Nearly all girls go through a phase when they feel like an "ugly duckling," especially in the middle-school years. Your teeth may seem too large for your face, your arms too long for your legs, and your eyelashes too stubby. Maybe you think you're too fat, too thin, too tall, or too short. Like we said, you're not alone. If you asked the most beautiful women in the world what they would change about themselves if they could, they'd all come up with something.

> It's very important to learn to like yourself-even your flaws. Growing up, I found that it's also important to be able to laugh at yourself and not take yourself too seriously.
> -Deborah

Don't wait on your body to change itself or to meet some strange set of beauty standards. You can begin to feel more beautiful, inside and out, right now. Try one or two of the following exercises:

1. ***Get up a half hour early*** tomorrow and take a walk outside. Think about the good things in your life, and thank God for them.

2. ***Buy a new perfume*** and enjoy it!

3. ***Spend part*** of your allowance on fresh flowers for your room (you can probably pick up a pretty bundle at the grocery store). Arrange them in a nice vase. If you really want a nice glow,

take flowers to a neighbor or a teacher.

4. *Take* a long bubble bath.

5. *Give* a friend an unexpected and sincere compliment. Or spend an hour helping an elderly neighbor with yard work.

6. *Write a paragraph* about what *beauty* means to you.

7. *Spend* at least fifteen minutes outside lying in the grass. Watch the clouds float by and find pictures in them.

8. *Wear a fresh* or silk flower in your hair or pinned to your shirt.

9. *Make a card* for someone special to say "Thank you for all you've done for me."

10. *Read a book* on something you've always wanted to learn about.

Did you notice something about the above list? Some suggestions are things that will help your *outer* beauty. But several others are ideas that will develop or encourage your *inner* beauty.

The Key to Inner Beauty

If you've followed all our suggestions and you still think beauty is beyond your grasp, there's one insight that will help you find inner beauty. You'll find it in Matthew 22:37-39:

> Jesus replied: "Love the Lord your God with all your heart and with all your soul and with all your mind. This is the first and greatest commandment. And the second is like it: 'Love your neighbor as yourself.'"

Jesus told us to love God with all our hearts, love others, and *love ourselves.* There's a difference between loving yourself in snobbish conceit and loving yourself the way Jesus intended. Conceited people see themselves as the center of the universe; they think they are better than everyone else. Jesus wants us to see ourselves as God sees us—we're precious, special to Him, and we're His children. When you realize how much God loves and *accepts* you, you are free to love yourself and others. That, above all, is the key to inner beauty.

What Guys Find Attractive

Angie polled a church group of teenage boys to find what they looked for in a girl. These guys, ages fourteen through seventeen, gave the results you might expect from teenage boys:

- ☐ 70 percent mentioned that a girl needed a "good body"
- ☐ 55 percent mentioned a "likeable personality"
- ☐ 35 percent mentioned "a pretty face"
- ☐ 10 percent said they wanted a "spiritual" girl

Pretty discouraging, huh? But then Angie polled a group of older Christian guys, eighteen through twenty-five, and got a totally different picture. The older guys agreed on five qualities an "ideal girl" must have, in the following order of importance:

1. Know Jesus Christ as Savior
2. Honest and sincere
3. Able to talk openly, a good communicator
4. Good self-image
5. Morally pure

Notice something? Although 70 percent of the younger guys mentioned a girl's physical attributes, a girl's physical beauty didn't make it into the top five list of the older guys. Maturity has a way of bringing things into perspective.

Both age groups of guys gave us a list of definite "turnoffs." What do they hate in a girl?

"Someone who doesn't talk."

"Arrogance, cockiness, and pretty girls who are stuck up."

"Girls who play mind games."

"Moodiness."

"Girls who talk only about themselves."

"Girls who act the way they think you want them to instead of just being themselves."

"Girls who fish for compliments by saying things like, 'I'm on a diet...' "

"Impatient girls."

"Girls who always want to know where they stand without ever just standing."

"Girls who wear too much makeup or jewelry."

"Girls who wear skimpy bathing suits, trying to show off their bodies."

"Girls who are smokers or drinkers."

Of course we can't promise that if you do the opposite of these things you'll turn into Miss Irresistible, but it doesn't hurt to know what bugs guys, does it? If you examine that "turn-off" list carefully, you'll see that guys really appreciate genuine interest, a girl who's not conceited, girls who are attractive from the inside out, and girls who are modest both in their attitudes and their dress.

Remember that some guys will hoot and whistle at girls who are immodest and dress to look "hot." If this is what you want, you'll always be able to find a bundle of male hormones seeking a temporary object of fulfillment. Be warned that this kind of attention, reputation, and relationship is destructive in the long run.

Beautiful Qualities

"Character contributes to beauty," Hollywood beauty Jacqueline Bisset told the *Los Angeles Times*. "It fortifies a woman as her youth fades. A mode of conduct, a standard of courage, discipline, fortitude, and integrity can do a great deal to make a woman beautiful."[5]

Leah Feldon, a noted fashion consultant and photo stylist, says, "While fashion changes from year to year, the words that are used to describe women of elegance have always remained constant: graceful, good-humored, kind, vital, determined, energetic, intelligent, and dedicated."[6]

There's more to being *graceful* than not tripping over your own feet. To be "full of grace" is to be kind, gentle, and generous, never panicking or being too worried about the small annoyances that come along. If your life is in God's hands, why should you worry? Allow God's grace to shine through you in your dealings with others.

Good humor means being optimistic and full of hope. If you're full of good humor, you won't be easily offended, nor will you go off and pout when someone accidentally or purposefully hurts your feelings. You'll be admired when you learn to hold your head high in confidence and good humor.

Vitality will make you fun to be around. Vitality means you have ideas, you're industrious, you're full of life, and eager to try new things. Maybe you're game to rent a pair of in-line skates for a trip across town. Of course your vitality won't lead you to do foolish things, because you're much too intelligent for that. Along with your vitality, you have a strong sense of self-control.

You can be filled with *determination* to see things through. You'll be dependable, and people know that you'll keep your promises and uphold your commitments. You'll be faithful.

You can be beautifully *energetic* in everything you do. You'll have a quick and ready smile, a twinkle in your eye, a spring in your step down the hall.

Intelligence is a quality of inner beauty. You don't have to be a National Honor Society member or a card-carrying genius, but you can be well-read and up on what's happening in the world. Read a book. Learn to care about what's going on outside your own neighborhood. Learn *how* to think, search out answers for your questions, and come up with and express your own opinions. You will be respected for it.

Dedication is our final quality of inner beauty. You are beautiful if you stand tall in the face of trouble. You are strong when you seek the truth and resolve never to settle for less than your best. You have the beauty of excellence when you dedicate yourself to treating the goofy kid from homeroom with the same grace and kindness you'd show to someone you really respect. Dedication is love in action.

These qualities of inner beauty are even more important than the benefits of having good hair, eyes, skin, and nails. Outer beauty fades with each passing year, but inner beauty grows more refined and more precious.

> The modeling business is filled with an emphasis on youth and superficial beauty. We all know that *everyone* will get old. If you are only concentrating on outer beauty, you will be disappointed. Inner beauty will last a lifetime. I like 2 Corinthians 4:16: "Therefore we do not lose heart. Though outwardly we are wasting away, yet inwardly we are being renewed day by day."
> -Wanda

In a moment we want you to put this book down and go to a mirror. Look carefully at yourself as if you were seeing yourself for the first time and decide which are your best physical attributes and which are your weakest. We've made suggestions about how to emphasize your good points and reduce the others, so decide for yourself that from this moment on, you're going to do your best to be your best.

But don't stop there. Still looking in your mirror, offer that reflection to God. Give yourself totally to the One who created you, and ask Him to make you beautiful on the inside. Ask God to teach you how to better love Him, love others, and love yourself as He does.

He will, you know, because it's on the *inside* that God can work to show His kindness through you to others. Other people may not remember your gorgeous eyes or the care with which you applied your makeup on a certain day, but they'll remember the kind words you gave or the hands you lent to help out in a crisis. They'll remember you for standing strong when others gave up. They'll be challenged by the attitudes and actions that reflect God's beauty, not by your looks!

That is the beauty we want you to find. That is the beauty that really counts.

Would you like to read about the difficulties some beautiful women faced? Older teens and adults should check out the **Dangerous Beauty Series** by Angela Hunt:

Esther: Royal Beauty
Bathsheba: Reluctant Beauty
Delilah: Treacherous Beauty (Spring 2016)

Available everywhere fine books are sold

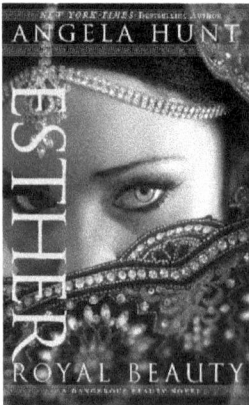

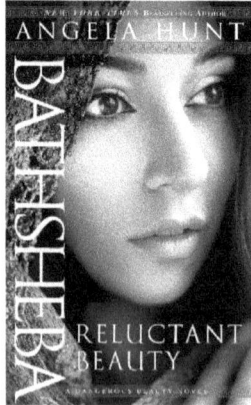

NOTES

Chapter 1: Hair—Your Crowning Glory

1. Martin Luther, *Table Talk,* quoted in *Dictionary of Quotations* (New York: Avenel Books, 1978), 297.
2. Louis Gignac, *Everything You Need to Know to Have Great-Looking Hair* (New York: The Viking Press, 1981).

Chapter 2: The Skin You're In

1. Stephen Petranek, "Get Smart. Get Scared. Get Out of the Sun," *Life,* August 1992, 56.

Chapter 3: The Eyes Have It!

1. Wilhelmina, *The New You* (Simon & Schuster).

Chapter 4: Makeup Magic

1. Heloise, *Heloise's Beauty Book* (New York: King Features Syndicate, Inc., Arbor House Publishing, 1985), 93.
2. Paula Begoun, *Blue Eyeshadow Should Be Illegal* (Seattle: Beginning Press, 1985).
3. Ibid.
4. Doug Peterson, "Is Christianity Only Meant for Beautiful Women?" *The Wittenburg Door,* August 1992, 28.

Chapter 5: Your Best Beauty Asset: Your Smile

1. David Lewis, *The Secret Language of Success* (New York: Carol and Graf Publishers, Inc., 1989), 68.
2. Jane Brody, *Jane Brody's The New York Times Guide to Personal Health* (New York: Times Books, 1982), 287.
3. Stephen Goodman quoted by Jane Brody, *Jane Brody's Guide,* 289.

Chapter 6: Sweet Feet and Fabulous Fingers

1. Elisa Ferri, Finger Tips (New York: Clarkson N. Pottler, Inc., 1988).

Chapter 7: Your Passion for Fashion

1. Carolyn Jabs, "Hate to See Yourself in a Bathing Suit? Here's How to Develop a Positive Body Image," *Lose Weight & Stay Healthy, Woman's Day Super Special,* Summer 1992,56. .
2. Trish Donnally, "New Bathing Suits Cut Shapely Figure," *St. Petersburg Times,* May 31, 1992.

Chapter 8: Fitness Fun

3.   Jane Brody, "Exercise for Children: Why and How to Start Young," *Jane Brody's The New York Times Guide to Personal Health* (New York: Times Books, 1982), 117.

4.   Natalie Angier, "Surprising Fact About Sleep," *Reader's Digest,* June 1991,33-34.

Chapter 9: Eating for Health and Beauty

1.   Dr. Charles Kuntzleman, "Eating Right: A Guide to Family Nutrition" (Arcadia, California: Focus on the Family Publishing, 1986), 3, 4.

2.   Irwin I. Lubowe, *M.D., A Teenage Guide to Healthy Skin and Hair* (New York: E.P. Dutton, 1979).

3.   Leroy R. Perry, Jr., "Are You Drinking Enough Water?" *Parade,* October22,1989,5.

4.   Ibid., 5.

5.   Carol Tavris, "Is Thin Still In?", *Woman's Day,* March 3,1987, 30.

6.   Dr. Reuben Andres quoted by Carol Tavris, ibid.

7.   Jennie Nash, "Diet Pills: Deadly?" *Seventeen,* March 1991,42.

8.   Geoffrey Cannon and Hetty Einzig, "Does Dieting Make You Fat?'*Reader's Digest,* November 1986,137.

9.   Doug Peterson, "Is Christianity Only Meant for Beautiful Women?" *The WittenburgFtoo Door,* August 1992,28.

10. Maureen Salaman, Foods *That Heal* (Menlo Park, California: Statford Publishing, 1989), 44.

11. Tacy Pullen, "The Dangers of Disorders," *Brio,* September 1992, 9.

Chapter 10: More Than Anything, Beauty Is an Attitude

1.   Carolyn Jabs, "Hate to See Yourself in a Bathing Suit? Here's How to Develop a Positive Body Image," *Lose Weight & Stay Healthy, Woman's Day Super Special,* Summer 1992,54.

2.   Ibid.

3.   Deutsche Presse Agentur, "Pageant Contestants Need to Show Inner Beauty, Too," *St. Petersburg Times,* August 6,1992,18A.

4.   Kaylan Pickford, *Always Beautiful* (New York: G.P. Putnam's Sons, 1985), 18.

5.   Jacqueline Bisset quoted in *The New York Times Public Library Book of 20th-century American Quotations* (New York: Warner Books, 1992), 99.

6.   Leah Feldon,D. *Dressing Rich* (New York: G.P. Putnam's Sons, 1982), 155.

ABOUT THE AUTHORS

Angela Hunt sang professionally and taught school before beginning her writing career. Since 1983, she has authored 125 books and over 700 magazine articles. Among her books are the award-winning *If I Had Long, Long Hair, The Tale of Three Trees,* and two series for teenagers: the *Cassie Perkins* series and the *Nicki Holland Mystery* series. She is very active in youth ministry with her husband. They live with their two mastiffs in the Tampa Bay area of Florida.

Laura Krauss Calenberg grew up tall and skinny. Schoolmates called her "Bean Pole" and "Daddy Long-legs," but she turned her height and frame into an advantage when at nineteen she began modeling in Paris. To date, she has graced the covers and pages of many international fashion magazines, appeared in numerous national ads and catalogs, and has been featured as a runway model in many top designer fashion shows around the world. Laura and her husband, Jeff (also a model), live in Florida and are represented there by two of the most prestigious modeling agencies in the world.

Although their careers require them to travel the globe, they have dedicated much of their time to establish IMPACT, a national nonprofit organization that unites young professionals to receive and extend God's love to the homeless, underprivileged, and needy in major cities.

www.ingramcontent.com/pod-product-compliance
Lightning Source LLC
Chambersburg PA
CBHW060504280326
41933CB00014B/2853